O A L
OXFORD ANAESTHESIA LIBRARY

Anaesthesia for Day Case Surgery

O A L

OXFORD ANAESTHESIA LIBRARY

Anaesthesia for Day Case Surgery

Jan Jakobsson, MD, PhD

Associate Professor
Karolinska Institutet,
Institution for Physiology and Pharmacology,
Department of Anaesthesia,
Foot and Ankle Surgical Center,
Stockholm,
Sweden

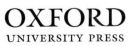
OXFORD
UNIVERSITY PRESS

OXFORD
UNIVERSITY PRESS

Great Clarendon Street, Oxford OX2 6DP

Oxford University Press is a department of the University of Oxford.
It furthers the University's objective of excellence in research, scholarship,
and education by publishing worldwide in

Oxford New York

Auckland Cape Town Dar es Salaam Hong Kong Karachi
Kuala Lumpur Madrid Melbourne Mexico City Nairobi
New Delhi Shanghai Taipei Toronto

With offices in

Argentina Austria Brazil Chile Czech Republic France Greece
Guatemala Hungary Italy Japan Poland Portugal Singapore
South Korea Switzerland Thailand Turkey Ukraine Vietnam

Oxford is a registered trade mark of Oxford University Press
in the UK and in certain other countries

Published in the United States
by Oxford University Press Inc., New York

British Library Cataloguing in Publication Data

Data available

Library of Congress Cataloging in Publication Data

Data available

Typeset by Newgen Imaging Systems (P) Ltd., Chennai, India
Printed in the UK
on acid-free paper by
Ashford Colour Press Ltd, Gosport, Hampshire.

ISBN 978–0–19–957713–2

10 9 8 7 6 5 4 3 2 1

Contents

Preface

Day case surgery is increasing worldwide. There are several reasons for the general trend towards reduced hospital stays and an increase in the number of ambulatory procedures. The economic benefit of the reduced number of hospital beds is one of the more powerful reasons. The introduction of new, less invasive surgical techniques, the advent of new short-acting anaesthetics and a better understanding of the physiology associated with surgical trauma are also of great importance. The increased understanding of the importance of the management of postoperative pain should not be neglected. The concept of multi-modal analgesia has to a major extent contributed to successful implementation of day surgery and is a simple and commonly used pain management strategy in day case surgery today.

Is there anything special about day case anaesthesia? Is there a need for special guidance? Day case surgery frequently involves elective, standardized, "high volume" procedures. The ultimate goals of day case surgery are to provide high-quality care and high patient turnover, an efficacious surgical production. In order to meet these goals, planning and logistics are of primary importance. Dedicated planning and trained/skilled personnel focused on not only on providing high quality of care but also patient turnover are basic and fundamental features of day case surgery. The anaesthesia service is one important part, but efficacious day surgery is a team effort.

Short stay in hospital, rapid mobilization and discharge, while important goals of day case surgery, need to be kept in perspective. It is of utmost importance to ensure that day surgery is safe and qualitatively equal to in-hospital surgery. Moving procedures from the in-hospital to the day case setting must not jeopardize safety and quality of care.

This pocketbook is intended to provide practical hands-on advice on the effective administration of day case anaesthesia in the adult patient. This pocketbook does not cover paediatric day case anaesthesia, which will be the focus of another volume in the series. The overall aim is to provide simple and pragmatic advice on how to set up, maintain and quality-assure efficacious day case anaesthesia routines. It supports the concept of simple, safe and efficacious anaesthesia titrated to each patient's unique intraoperative needs in combination with balanced analgesia or so called "multi-modal pain management". This pocketbook was not designed to provide detailed information about the skills and techniques needed to perform nerve blocks, however, it does strongly promote the use of local anaesthesia wherever possible. This includes the use of local infiltration, intra-articular injected, peripheral blocks and, when applicable, regional blocks; single injections as well as continuous infusion als after discharge and "home-pump systems".

The aims of this pocketbook are to:

- address special features and demands associated with day case anaesthesia;
- provide suggestions on the optimal process of converting from in-hospital to day case routines;
- provide tips about how to set up a "new" hospital-based or freestanding day case service.

Readers are strongly recommended to use this book as a starting point rather than as a definitive guide to day case anaesthesia. It is hoped that clinicians and those interested in setting up a day case service will find it helpful in gaining success with their day case programmes.

Jan Jakobsson
Stockholm,
Sweden

Abbreviations

ACE	angiotensin-converting enzyme
ASA	American Society of Anesthesiologists
CFU	colony forming units
CNS	central nervous system
CXR	chest X-ray
COPA	cuffed oropharyngeal airway
D & C	dilatation and curettage
ECG	electrocardiogram
EMLA	eutectic mixture of local anaesthetic
FBC	full blood count
GKI	glucose potassium and insulin
GP	General Practitioner
I-Gel	intersurgical airway
INR	international normalized ratio
IVRA	intravenous regional anaesthesia
KC1	potassium chloride
LAVH	laparoscopic assisted vaginal hysterectomy
LMA	laryngeal mask airway
m/r	modified release
NNT	needed to treat
no per os	nothing to be taken orally
NSAID	non-steroidal anti-inflammatory drugs
OCPS	oral contraceptive pills
OR	operating room
PACU	post-anaesthetic care unit
PCI	percutaenous cardiac interventions
PCRA	patient-controlled regional analgesia
PDNV	post-discharge nausea and vomiting
PONV	postoperative nausea and vomiting
SLIPA	streamlined liner of the pharynx airway

TCI	target control infusion system
TIVA	total intravenous anaesthesia
TOF	train of four ratio
TWA	time weighted average
VAS	visual analogue scale
VIMA	volatile inaduction and maintenance of anaesthesia

x

Chapter 1

Day surgery, ambulatory anaesthesia, and office-based procedures

Key points

- Day surgery—admission to and discharge from the hospital on the day of surgery–is becoming increasingly popular. An anaesthetic service should provide effective and safe intraoperative as well as postoperative course, but should also ascertain if the patient is safe to discharge within hours after the end of surgery/ anaesthesia.
- Building a day surgical programme involves all stakeholders and should focus on providing the patient with dedicated and efficient care still taking all national set regulations and guidelines into account. The mind-set and multi-disciplinary involvement of the unit is of outmost importance for successful implementation.
- All personnel should be involved and engaged in building a patient-focused production-oriented logistic programme.

1.1 Some basic definitions

Discharge from hospital on the day of surgery is generally referred to as **day case surgery**. There are, however, several synonyms for day surgery, and the exact definition may differ between institutions as well as between countries. The terms **outpatient surgery, ambulatory surgery, day case surgery, same day surgery**, and **office-based surgery**, all refer to similar concepts. Avoiding the traditional in-hospital stay is a shared objective of these various concepts. In some countries, ambulatory surgery may include a one-night in-hospital stay or a stay in close proximity to the hospital (e.g., a hospital attached hotel).

The number of day case procedures performed is increasing and more procedures are now being transferred from in-hospital care to short-stay programmes. Additionally more complex procedures are now frequently performed as ambulatory surgery. Older and more fragile patients are also more frequently scheduled for day case surgery. In some countries, a majority of surgical procedures are now performed as ambulatory surgery; however, there are still hug differences between countries (see Table 1.1) (http://iaas-med.com/modules/content/survey2005.pdf).

Far more surgical specialities now perform day case surgery to some extent. Eye surgery, plastic surgery, and hand surgery are today performed predominantly as ambulatory surgery. The mindset of day case anaesthesia is also very much the same for all kinds of office-based procedures that require deep sedation/anaesthesia. A similar anaesthetic approach is commonly applied for a variety of diagnostic and interventional procedures in radiology departments, catheterization-labs, and endoscopic units.

There are many reasons behind the trend to reduce the in-hospital stay associated with surgery. New surgical techniques have had a major impact and, in particular, minimally invasive techniques have made huge contribution. A better understanding of the pathophysiology associated with surgical trauma has also had an impact. Early mobilization and enteral feeding is beneficial in most procedures and it has been shown not to impair safety, and in fact has been shown to reduce the risk for thrombo-embolic complications and gastrointestinal translocation-related infections. Reducing the in-hospital stay

Country	Endoscopic sterilization	Legal abortion	D&C	LAVH	Cysto/ rectocele
Australia	83.4	90.0	81.5	0.2	2.3
Belgium	57.8	—	80.9	0.1	4.1
Denmark	90.6	97.3	91.3	4.4	8.4
England	80.8	62.0	78.8	1.0	1.2
Finland	70.2	85.7	55.6	0.4	2.1
France	10.4	83.5	49.9	0.2	2.9
Germany	10.6	16.5	77.7	0.2	38.6
Hong Kong	—	—	—	—	—
Italy	28.9	84.4	39.5	1.4	1.24
Veneto reg.	51.8	96.4	70.4	0.5	3.0
Netherlands	92.0	89.4	71.7	0	0.5
Norway	11.2	97.0	65.8	0.9	3.5
Portugal	28.8	—	21.8	0	0.2
Scotland	79.0	76.8	68.7	0.2	2.0
Spain	67.9	21.4	22.4	0	1.0
Sweden	82.2	92.1	66.2	1.4	7.8
USA	90.3	84.2	85.1	3.1	25.7

Table 1.1 Percentage of gynaecological procedures performed as ambulatory surgery

Table 1.1 is reproduced with permission from IAAS © 2005.

also reduces the risk of nosocomial infections. For children and older patients, the return to the home environment may indeed result in psychological benefits and may reduce the risk for anxiety and fear associated with the hospital visit and for the elderly risk of cognitive deterioration.

New drugs, anaesthetics, and analgesics with rapid onset and offset of action for intra-operative use have improved the recovery process. The introduction of dedicated programmes taking all aspects of the perioperative course into account is, however, perhaps the most important change. The multi-disciplinary approach has had a major impact on day surgery, and structured and well-described planning (i.e., who does what and when) is one of most important factors determining success. The mindset of the multi-disciplinary team—creating devoted team spirit and clear process-oriented goals among all personnel involved, including the surgeon—is of utmost importance.

Also, major surgical procedures have been shown to be reassuringly safe when performed as day case or short stay procedures when adopting strict dedicated programmes and, of course, with the involvement of a skilled and motivated responsible surgeon. Recently, reports of successful day case disc hernia resection and short-stay bariatric surgery have been published. These reports highlight the importance of proper patient selection and preparation. However a dedicated anaesthetic regimen together with experienced surgeons in high-volume centres seems to be among the main criteria for success.

1.2 How much day surgery?

When figures and results are discussed it should be acknowledged that in Europe clinicians often refer to day case surgery (i.e., the patient is admitted and discharged on the day of surgery); however, in some countries, ambulatory surgery includes one-night stay and discharge within 24 hours. For further national definitions see http://iaas-med.com/modules/content/Acr977.tmp.pdf. Differences in the amount of ambulatory surgical procedures is shown in Table 1.2.

The reported number of all procedures performed in the day case surgery setting will also vary depending on whether office-based procedures (e.g. gastroscopies, colonoscopies and other endoscopic procedures performed under "sedation") are included or not.

1.3 Day surgical unit/department/centre

The unit itself should also be considered. The day case surgical unit may be part of an ordinary operating department, or rather a unit within a hospital with all multi-disciplinary resources available and the

Table 1.2 Percentage of general surgical procedures performed as ambulatory surgery

Country	Breast excision	Mastec- tomy	Lap. Chol.	Anti-reflux surg.	Haemorrhoi- dectomy
Australia	57.5	1.5	1.9	0.5	70.7
Belgium	—	—	1.3	0.2	32.0
Denmark	43.4	8.3	25.6	9.0	86.7
England	33.5	2.3	6.5	2.6	67.3
Finland	25.8	2.9	17.3	2.7	34.4
France	13.5	4.5	0.3	0.2	5.7
Germany	52.1	13.6	unknown	1.9	39.7
Hong Kong	—	—	5.4	—	29.2
Italy	70.2	1.9	2.8	1.0	23.9
Veneto reg.	92.1	0.8	0.5	0.5	59.5
Netherlands	0.9	0.7	3.5	1.7	65.7
Norway	44.1	16.6	17.4	7.9	64.5
Portugal	33.1	0.4	1.9	0.2	—
Scotland	62.7	1.5	1.4	0	72.9
Spain	42.7	1.3	6.1	2.9	35.3
Sweden	45.5	7.8	14.3	2.5	87.2
USA	98.3	63.5	52.0	2.1	96.2

Table 1.2 is reproduced with permission from IAAS © 2005.

option to keep the patient if deemed necessary. It may, on the other hand, be a freestanding day surgical unit without the in-hospital facilities in close proximity. Small office-based surgical centres are increasingly popular in some countries. The physical distance and the collaboration with an emergency hospital are of importance. In complicated cases referral must be acceptably safe.

All of these aspects should be taken into account when the day surgical programme is to be instituted. The day surgical programme should offer efficacious patient turnover but without jeopardizing safety or quality of care.

1.4 **Medicolegal aspects**

Day surgical anaesthesia should follow all national standards and guidelines. The unit and the programme should apply to the same principals and safety considerations as for regular in-hospital care.

- Fasting routines should be fully adhered to in accordance with general national without food or drink (*no per os*) guidelines.
- National programmes/guidelines for thrombo-prophyalxis, blood-borne infections, and multi-resistant bacteria should be adhered to.

Many decisions include both anaesthetic and surgical considerations. The unit must develop clear routines, that are well structured and that allow for transparency of decisions processes associated with care of the day surgical patient.

Responsibilities should be clearly and explicitly established all the way through from: identification of patient, control of surgical site, taking away intravenous lines, before discharge, to prescription routines. Prescription and information about pain medication should be explicitly stated. Decision about when thromboprophylaxis should be given and prescription of anticoagulants to take at home should also be clear. Standard operating procedures for the entire hospital care process are of huge value and are strongly recommended.

1.5 Information: a key obligation

All patients should be carefully informed prior to surgery. Providing the patient with information about the entire perioperative course is of utmost importance, and should include details of pain management, how to mobilize, general wound care, and rehabilitation. Both written and oral information should be provided and patients should receive appropriate information regarding any unanticipated complications, including severe postoperative pain. It is mandatory that patients understand and are able to follow given instructions and that they give their full consent to the scheduled procedure and care within the frame of the day case programme. The option of web sites and videos for information regarding both specific procedures and the general programme should be considered. A web site that can be easily updated and is easily accessible for patients and relatives can be a useful educational aid.

Another current trend in clinical practice is for some typical day case procedures to be performed as office-based procedures with only limited anaesthetist support. Non-anaesthetist sedation is increasingly discussed. Office-based minor superficial surgery has commonly been performed under local anaesthesia in most hospitals for decades. There has also been a long history of surgeons providing their patients with small amounts of opioid analgesics and or anxiolytics prior to painful procedures.

1.6 Sedation and analgesia with limited anaesthetist support

1.6.1 Pre-mixed nitrous oxide and oxygen 50% vol. each

Various forms of analgesia/sedation have been used in endoscopy units and other office based settings in order to facilitate performance and reduce procedural pain. Entonox® is the registered trademark of

BOC Healthcare for a medical gas mixture of 50% nitrous oxide and 50% oxygen and has a very long and most reassuring safety record for procedural pain management in children as well as in adults. The fixed concentration of 50% vol. of nitrous oxide and 50% vol. of oxygen guarantees appropriate inspired oxygen concentration. The 50% nitrous oxide provides analgesia and relaxation but rarely causes loss of consciousness. The fixed gas mixture is administered by inhalation and is thus non-invasive. For the "self-controlled mode of administration—patient controlled analgesia", the patient should be instructed how to hold and use the mask and how to breath from the demand valve. Requiring the patient to hold the mask tight and breathe normally himself provides unique safety features. The demand valve does not open if the mask is not kept tight and subsequently the inspiration efforts give rise to a negative pressure of 2–4 cm H_2O, minimizing the risk of over sedation and associated depression of security reflexes, therefore minimizing the risk for respiratory depression and regurgitation/aspiration. Working with nitrous oxide should, of course, follow set national recommendations regarding the workplace environment. Ventilation should be adequate so as to avoid high ambient air-trace concentrations.

1.6.2 **Oral benzodiazepines and topical anaesthesia**

Oral benzodiazepines (e.g. midazolam) are a non-invasive alternative. Midazolam oral liquid is absorbed rapidly via the buccal route and may be an option to reduce perioperative anxiety. The use of midazolam administered nasally has been described in children, but the experience in adults is limited.

Topical local anaesthesia should not be forgotten and can be clinically useful as many patients fear needles. Topical anaesthesia and eutectic mixture of local anaesthetic (EMLA®) (http://www1.astrazeneca-us.com/pi/EMLA.pdf) have been shown to be effective in children and should also be seen as an option in adults with needle phobia. There is also the new option of local anaesthesia plaster Rapydan® (EUSA Pharma; http://www.eusapharma.com/rapydan.html) that develops some warmth providing a more rapid onset and also a vasodilatation potentially making the cannulation easier in adults as well as in children.

1.6.3 **Intravenous sedation and analgesia in the office-based setting**

The huge expansion of office-based surgery, as well as other diagnostic and therapeutic minimally invasive procedures has increased the demand for sedation, anxiolysis, and analgesia. The request profile is for a rapid onset of action as well as a rapid offset of action, in other words a fast-acting sedative/analgesic that wears off quickly after the procedure leaving the patient alert once again. The intravenous route and the usage of fast-acting sedatives and/or analgesics ave become of increased interest. In many countries and institutions there is insufficient anaesthesia staff to cope with this increased demand. Intravenous "sedation" performed using drugs such as propofol, midazolam, alfenatil, and fentanyl is increasingly common.

Today general European guidelines on non-anaesthetist sedation are available. These general guidelines must be adopted and accepted locally and the importance of avoiding deeper sedation must be strongly emphasized. Non-anaesthetists sedation should only include drugs and doses in order to **reduce anxiety and apprehension** but **maintain consciousness and spontaneous breathing**—so called conscious sedation. For deeper sedation and analgesia, whenever loss of consciousness and protecting reflexes may be anticipated, ordinary general anaesthesia routines should be followed. Deeper levels of sedation should be administered following the same routines as for general anaesthesia under the control of an anaesthetist.

1.6.4 **In minor procedures**

There are strict general guidelines on sedation and analgesia for minor procedures without the surveillance of an anaesthetist. These general guidelines are based on the level of sedation and associated degree of depression of vital functions including protective reflexes. The sedation levels have been defined as follows:

- **Sedation level 1**: Fully awake.
- **Sedation level 2**: Drowsy.
- **Sedation level 3**: Apparently asleep but arousable by normal speech.
- **Sedation level 4**: Apparently asleep but responding to a standardized physical stimulus, such as glabellar tap trapezius squeezes.
- **Sedation level 5**: Asleep, but not responding to physical stimuli (comatose). This state is similar or synonymous with anaesthesia.

Sedation and/or analgesia techniques performed by non-anaesthetist clinicians are not reasonably expected to result in such a level of sedation that the vital, protective reflexes are lost.

In order to allow patients to undergo unpleasant procedures, the objective of sedation and/or analgesia by non-anaesthetists is to achieve a level of sedation comparable to "sedation level 2 or 3" using appropriate pharmacological techniques.

In relation to the serious risks associated with "sedation level 4 (or even 5)", this level of sedation is only to be handled by trained, adequately skilled clinicians under the control of an anaesthetist.

Intravenous sedation with propofol and propofol opiate combination without anaesthetist surveillance is still controversial. Non-anaesthetist sedation must be accepted nationally and adopted locally. Written procedures should be in place and signed off by the responsible physician.

1.7 Documentation and records

An accurate anaesthesia record is mandatory for all day case anaesthetic procedures. The anaesthesia record should follow the national standard for anaesthetic records and be stored accordingly. In order to document and retrieve any sedation, the sedative course should be recorded in an ordinary anaesthetic record where vital signs including level of sedation should be recorded in a timely manner.

Further reading

Bergland A, Gislason H, Raeder J. Fast-track surgery for bariatric laparoscopic gastric bypass with focus on anaesthesia and peri-operative care. Experience with 500 cases. *Acta Anaesthesiol Scand.* 2008 Nov; **52**(10): 1394–9.

Canet J, Raeder J, Rasmussen LS, Enlund M, Kuipers HM, Hanning CD, Jolles J, Korttila K, Siersma VD, Dodds C, Abildstrom H, Sneyd JR, Vila P, Johnson T, Muñoz Corsini L, Silverstein JH, Nielsen IK, Moller JT; ISPOCD2 investigators. Cognitive dysfunction after minor surgery in the elderly. *Acta Anaesthesiol Scand.* 2003 Nov; **47**(10): 1204–10.

Knape JT, Adriaensen H, van Aken H, Blunnie WP, Carlsson C, Dupont M, Pasch T; Board of Anaesthesiology of the European Union of Medical Specialists. Guidelines for sedation and/or analgesia by non-anaesthesiology doctors. *Eur J Anaesthesiol.* 2007 Jul; **24**(7): 563–7.

Raeder J. Bariatric procedures as day/short stay surgery: is it possible and reasonable? *Curr Opin Anaesthesiol.* 2007 Dec; **20**(6): 508–12. Review.

Chapter 2

Anaesthesia equipment and monitoring in day surgery anaesthesia

Key points

- Day case anaesthesia and office-based anaesthesia should be performed with adequate delivery and monitoring equipment in accordance with national guidelines.
- All equipment and monitoring devices should be checked on a regular basis and control of function is mandatory before administration of each anaesthetic.
- A simple checklist should be followed before each procedure, ensuring proper function of equipment, control of patient identification and procedure (site of surgery should be marked by the responsible surgeon).
- Day case anaesthesia should have the same form of safety and risk management system as in-hospital care.
- Control of equipment, preoperative assessment, intraoperative, and postoperative observations should be documented and stored in accordance to regulations.
- Ventilation of the operating theatre should be in accordance with national regulations and adjusted in order to minimize the risk for contamination. Scavenging of waste gas should also adhere to national guidelines. Work-place air quality, concentrations of trace concentration of waste anaesthetics, pollutants from diathermia or use of chemicals in the wound, and measured colony forming units (CFU) should be in accordance with national guidelines.
- There should be a system in place for incident and failure reporting. Failures and incidents should be analyzed and the analysis should communicated within the unit in order to avoid reoccurrence.

2.1 **Safety first**

Anaesthesia for day surgery should be performed in accordance with both basic and general roles and routines. Day case anaesthesia has been shown to be reassuringly safe when performed according to conventional hospital standards. Studies of major morbidity as well as the need for return to hospital following day case anaesthesia have not shown reasons for any major concern.

In a classic paper, Warner *et al.* looked at a total of 38,598 patients aged 18 years and older undergoing 45,090 consecutive ambulatory procedures and anaesthetics. Contact rates for 72 hours and 30 days were 99.94% and 95.9%, respectively. Overall morbidity and mortality rates were very low. In all, 14 patients had myocardial infarction (1:3220), seven had a central nervous system deficit (1:6441), five had pulmonary embolism (1:9018), and five had respiratory failure (1:9018). Four events (13%) occurred within eight hours of surgery (1:11,273), 15 (48%) in the next 40 hours (1:3006), and 12 (39%) in the next 28 days (1:3758).

A later study from Denmark reviewed two centres and a total of 16,048 patients that underwent 18,736 day surgery procedures including 4,829 surgical abortions. The study analyzed the 18,736 procedures for subsequent contact wtih Danish hospitals within 60 post-operative days, and the associated morbidity and mortality. The study showed that the day surgery procedures resulted in very low morbidity. Altogether no incidences of myocardial infarction, central nervous system deficit, pneumonia, or death were recorded that could definitely or likely be attributed to day surgery.

We must, however, keep in mind that these reports describe the outcomes after day surgery in the United States 20 years ago and in Denmark almost 10 years ago, respectively. More and more complex procedures are today being performed as day surgery, and more elderly patients and patients with co-morbidity are seen on a day case basis. Close follow-up and incident reporting in order to learn and improve performance should be a natural part of the day surgical programme (see also chapter 9).

2.2 **Anaesthetic equipment and maintenance**

The anaesthetic machine should comply with set national standards and ordinary resuscitation equipment should be readily available. Anaesthesia equipment standards should be identical to those for in-patient anaesthesia. The anaesthetic workstation used may, however, have fewer technical features (e.g. invasive pressure monitoring, sophisticated ventilator modes, and sophisticated monitoring such as pressure volume loop are not needed for basic day case anaesthesia).

The anaesthetic machine does not need to be an expensive full anaesthetic work station but the basic components for anaesthesia should comply with set standards. The anaesthetic equipment can be adapted to the individual procedures performed (e.g., a ventilator may not be necessary in providing anaesthesia to spontaneously breathing patients only).

The operating table should comply with standards; it should be easy to change the position of the table, tilt the patient's head down and raise the legs if necessary.

Equipment for intubation should be readily available and checked at least once daily.

Also, recovery facilities must comply with accepted standards but may be adapted to the caseload.

In order to facilitate patient turn over it is of value to have both a traditional recovery area, recovery room with oxygen, and vital sign monitoring as well as stage 2 recovery where patients are encouraged to start to ambulate, drink, and get ready for discharge.

Storage of drugs and medications should comply with set standards. Cupboards and refrigerators for medications should be constructed and provide temperatures in accordance with recommendations For drugs classed as narcotics records should be available for registration in accordance with national and local regulations.

Cleaning routines, availability of disposables, syringes, needles, etc. should follow strict written routines.

There should be a written and regularly rehearsed rescue plan, for use in situations of failed intubation, anaphylaxis, and cardiac emergencies—cardiac arrest or severe circulatory failure. Emergency equipment and plans for resuscitation, including a defibrillator, should be readily available in close proximity to the operating theatre as well the recovery area.

An emergency plan in the event of fire, including emergency evacuation of patients, should be available.

2.3 Monitoring equipment

Monitoring equipment intraoperatively should include classic vital sign monitoring:

- heart rate—must;
- blood pressure—must;
- respiratory rate—must.

It should also include:

- pulse oximetry—must;
- ECG is strongly recommended but may be optional in healthy ASA scale 1 patients followed by pulse oximetry;

- on-line gas monitoring:
  - FiO_2—must
  - $EtCO_2$—must
  - end tidal anaesthetic gas concentration—strongly recommended.

Also strongly recommended:
  - non-invasive automatic blood pressure monitoring device with memory and trend;
  - SpO_2 wave form and trend analysis;
  - inspiratory gas concentrations.

2.3.1 **Neuromuscular monitoring**

Neuromuscular monitoring is mandatory in all cases where muscle relaxation is used in order to monitor the effect of the neuromuscular block and the full reversal before awakening.

2.3.2 **Nice to have**

Brain monitoring, **anaesthetic depth monitor**, BIS or Entropy, adds additional information but is optional (see also chapter on anaesthetic drugs and PONV)

A target control infusion system (TCI) for delivery of propofol and remifentanil improves drug delivery of total intravenous anaesthesia.

2.3.3 **Scavenging: workplace ambient air control**

In operating theatres where inhaled anaesthetics are used, a scavenging device should be available in order to secure the health of staff. Ambient air-trace concentrations and time weighted average (TWA) values of inhaled anaesthetics should comply with set national guidelines. Forced ventilation in order to reduce wound contamination is standard in most countries and guidelines should be followed and checked accordingly.

2.4 **The recovery area**

The recovery area should include equipment for monitoring of vital signs:
  - heart rate (pulse oximetry);
  - blood pressure;
  - oxygen saturation;
  - body temperature.

Equipment for administration of oxygen, oxygen supplementation, and for suctioning must be available. There should be ECG monitoring when needed and rescue equipment should be available.

Vital signs, level of consciousness, VAS for pain, and medications should be recorded in accordance with set routines.

Many day case patients already regain consciousness and are fully awake in theatre. These patients may be **fast-tracked, bypassing the recovery room and transferred to the stage 2 recovery area directly.** Also, these patients should, of course, be observed during the early stage following the end of anaesthesia with regard to alertness, pain, and eventual fatigue/emesis.

2.4.1 **Medicinal gases**

Oxygen, medical air, and suction equipment should be available with back up as appropriate. Gas sources and suction equipment should be checked once daily. Tubes and connections should be checked prior to each procedure.

Oxygen should be readily available. Most hospitals have a central pip-system that is kept under the control of skilled medicinal technicians. In minor surgical centres, oxygen availability must be secured from local oxygen storage or oxygen central.

Oxygen may be produced at site with an oxygenator. In such cases it should be acknowledged that the oxygen concentration usually amounts to approximately 90–94 % and inert gases, especially argon, are present in an increased concentration and may accumulate if low flow in a circle system is used. Monitoring of FiO_2 and oxygen saturation should, of course, be carried out in order to secure proper oxygenation.

Back-up oxygen in cylinders must be available in case of a device shutdown.

Compressed air should be available for medical use. Medicinal air for use as part of the fresh gas flow must be available. Compressed air for suction devices and medical devices should be readily available.

Nitrous oxide is optional. The well-acknowledged additive effects between nitrous oxide and inhaled as well as intravenous anaesthetics should be considered. When available from a hospital system or cylinder, nitrous oxide, as part of the fresh gas, adds speed and cost-effectiveness. When starting a new unit, investment must be balanced against the benefit and cost savings from its use.

2.5 **Technical support and surveillance**

A structured protocol for cleaning, maintenance, and calibration of monitoring equipment should be at hand.

A proactive control system for service in accordance with Users Manuals covering all technical equipment should be in place.

Reporting of failures and incidents should also be a natural part of the programme in order to repair faulty equipment and evaluate whether improvements in use and handling can avoid reoccurrence.

13

Box 2.1 Summary tips for setting up a day case anaesthesia service: anaesthesia equipment and monitoring

Special demands

No—safe and efficacious machines and equipment in accordance with accepted national standards and regulations.

Converting

Equipment used for in-hospital anaesthesia is more than suitable for day case anaesthesia.

Setting up

Anaesthesia and monitoring equipment should comply with set national recommendations and guidelines.

Think about

Equipment should be functional and adhere to set standards, however there may not be any need for complex or sophisticated devices as long as safety and functionality is secured.

Further reading

Engbaek J, Bartholdy J, Hjortsø NC. Return hospital visits and morbidity within 60 days after day surgery: a retrospective study of 18,736 day surgical procedures. *Acta Anaesthesiol Scand.* 2006 Sep; **50**(8): 911–9.

Mangram AJ, Horan TC, Pearson ML, Silver LC, Jarvis WR. Guideline for Prevention of Surgical Site Infection, 1999. Centers for Disease Control and Prevention (CDC) Hospital Infection Control Practices Advisory Committee. *Am J Infect Control.* 1999 Apr; **27**(2): 97–132.

Mérat F, Mérat S. Occupational hazards related to the practice of anaesthesia. *Ann Fr Anesth Reanim.* 2008 Jan; **27**(1): 63–73. Review.

Parker CJ, Snowdon SL. Predicted and measured oxygen concentrations in the circle system using low fresh gas flows with oxygen supplied by an oxygen concentrator. *Br J Anaesth.* 1988 Oct; **61**(4): 397–402.

Warner MA, Shields SE, Chute CG. Major morbidity and mortality within 1 month of ambulatory surgery and anesthesia.. *JAMA.* 1993 Sep 22–29; **270**(12): 1437–41.

Chapter 3

Patient selection and preparation for day surgical procedures

Key points

- The day case patient must be discharged from hospital care within hours after the end of anaesthesia; thus special attention must be given to proper patient selection, preparation, and information.
- All patients scheduled for day case anaesthesia should be assessed preoperatively and reviewed for risk factors prior to the start of anaesthesia
- Preoperative questionnaires that can be filled in by the patient before coming to hospital are often of great help and can help facilitate the assessment process.
- Information (oral and, whenever feasible, written) regarding the anaesthesia administered and the post-operative course including pain management should be provided and signed by responsible anaesthetist.
- Patients should give informed consent.
- Routine preoperative testing is not mandatory in the typical case on ASA scale 1–2 patients; preoperative investigations and tests should be performed on an individual basis on the information retrieved during the preoperative assessment.
- Preparation and information should be provided well in advance in order to avoid late cancellation or delays.
- Planning of the "list for the day" should be done on the basis of preoperative information about the patient, taking into account the type of procedure and eventual special needs (e.g. position, equipment, etc.).
- Well-informed and motivated patients help to facilitate rapid patient turnover.

3.1 **Preoperative assessment**

Day surgery commonly involves minor and intermediate surgical procedures (e.g., arthroscopy, open hernia repair, and "minor" laparoscopic procedures) typically performed in healthy ASA scale 1–2 patients. Preoperative assessment should still be done in each individual case. Much of the basic information can, however, be obtained by way of a patient questionnaire or from an interview with a nurse. Nonetheless, each patient scheduled to undergo anaesthesia/ sedation should have been evaluated and assessed prior to induction (http://student.bmj.com/issues/07/01/education/12.php).

All patients should be assessed in order to ascertain the following:

- General health (including smoking/nicotine habits misuse/abuse, chronic infections).
- An assessment of functional capacity (see Table 3.1).
- Regular medications (hormones and OCPs).
- History of any allergic reactions and or adverse drug reactions.
- Prior anaesthetic experience (including PONV, bleeding, or thrombo-embolic complications).
- Last intake of food and fluids.

Each patient should be assigned an ASA physical status scale class and an anaesthetic prescription. Anaesthesia may be mostly standardized, but all patients should still have been prescribed an individual plan for the intraoperative as well as the early postoperative period. Preoperative information as well as prescribed handling, drugs/technique, etc. should be documented and available although the hospital course. Figure 3.1 shows a grid of anaesthetic and surgical risk.

Major morbidity and mortality following ambulatory surgery is exceedingly low. Minor adverse cardiac events during the intraoperative period are associated with hypertension and the elderly. Minor adverse respiratory events during the intraoperative period are

Table 3.1 Functional capacity expressed in metabolic equivalents	
Metabolic equivalents (METs)	**Physical activity**
1–4	Eating, dressing, dishwashing, and walking around the house
4–10	Climbing a flight of stairs, walking on level ground at >6 km/hr, running briefly, playing golf
>10	Strenuous sports: swimming, singles tennis, football

Table 3.1 is reproduced from *Oxford Handbook of Anaesthesia, Second Edition*, edited by Keith G. Allman and Iain H. Wilson, (2006), with permission from Oxford University Press.

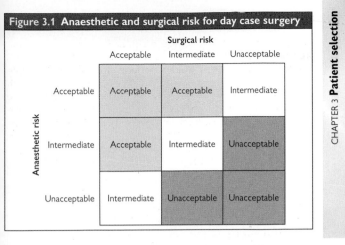

Figure 3.1 Anaesthetic and surgical risk for day case surgery

		Surgical risk	
	Acceptable	Intermediate	Unacceptable
Acceptable	Acceptable	Acceptable	Intermediate
Intermediate	Acceptable	Intermediate	Unacceptable
Unacceptable	Intermediate	Unacceptable	Unacceptable

Anaesthetic risk

associated with obesity. Respiratory events during the postoperative period are associated with obesity, smoking, and asthma. Prolonged stays following ambulatory surgery are predominantly caused by surgical factors or minor symptoms such as pain or nausea. Surgical factors are also the main causes of unplanned admissions. Patients older than 85 years of age, significant co-morbidity, and multiple admissions to hospital in the six months preceding ambulatory surgery, however, are all associated with higher re-admission rates. Table 3.2 and Figure 3.2 show rates of adverse events in the operating theatre.

3.1.1 The ASA scale 2–3 patient

ASA scale 2–3 patients with well-controlled cardiovascular, pulmonary, or endocrine disease may of course also be eligible for day surgery. These patients should be assessed preoperatively in accordance with set routines. Medical history, medication, allergy, and previous anaesthetic experience should be evaluated. Assessment of physical capacity, ability to walk on flat ground, walk up-hill, and climb stairs is an easy way to get a basic evaluation of their physical reserves. Wherever necessary, consultation with the general practitioner or specialist taking regular care of the patient should be initiated. The ASA scale 2–3 patient should be optimized prior to surgery.

Table 3.2 Association between pre-existing medical conditions and adverse outcomes

Medical condition	Associated adverse outcome
Congestive heart failure	12% prolongation of postoperative stay
Hypertension	two-fold increase in the risk of intraoperative cardiovascular events
Asthma	five-fold increase in the risk of postoperative respiratory events
Smoking	four-fold increase in the risk of postoperative respiratory events
Obesity	four-fold increase in the risk of intraoperative and postoperative respiratory events
GE reflux	eight-fold increase in the risk of intubation-related adverse events

GE = gastroesophageal

Table 3.2 is reproduced from Bryson *et al.* (2004) Patient selection in ambulatory anaesthesia: An evidence-based review: Part I. *Can J Anaesth* **51**(8): 768–81, with permission from Springer–Verlag.

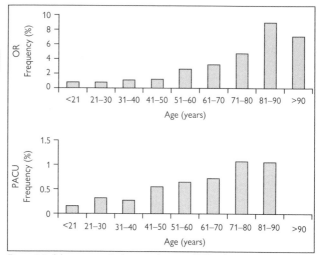

Figure 3.2 Adverse events in the operating room (OR) and post-anaesthesia care unit (PACU) with increasing age. Reproduced from Bryson *et al.* (2004) Patient selection in ambulatory anaesthesia: An evidence-based review: Part I. *Can J Anaesth* **51**(8): 768–81, with permission from Springer–Verlag.

Table 3.3 Cardiological referral					
Exercise tolerance	Any	<4 METs	>4 METs	<4 METs	>4 METs
Surgical risk	Cardiac Major	Risk Inter-mediate		Minor	
High	Refer	Refer	Refer	Refer	Operate
Intermediate	Refer	Refer	Operate	Operate	Operate
Low	Refer	Operate	Operate	Operate	Operate

Table 3.3 is reproduced from *Oxford Handbook of Anaesthesia, Second Edition*, edited by Keith G. Allman and Iain H. Wilson, (2006), with permission from Oxford University Press.

3.1.2 Regular medications

Regular medications should be recorded and, if necessary, adjusted prior to surgery. Most regular medications can, however, be kept. Recently the suitability of beta-blockers and ACE inhibitors has been discussed, however at present no consensus has been reached regarding whether stopped or their continued use.

3.1.3 Antiplatelet therapy

The risks versus benefits of regular anti platelet therapy must be evaluated individually in each patient. The maintenance or withdrawal of anti platelet therapy is a decision that includes both anaesthetic and surgical considerations. The decision to stop or continue must be settled by a firm and structured interaction between the surgeon and the anaesthetist.

Many ambulatory surgical procedures present low bleeding risk. The current attitude in this setting is to maintain aspirin therapy and possibly other anti platelet drugs throughout the perioperative period.

Special attention should be given in a procedure with an increased risk associated with bleeding. Sensitive markers of platelet function demonstrate increased bleeding tendency for several days after withdrawal of aspirin therapy and thus support discontinuation of aspirin therapy five days before elective surgery (with the operation being performed on the sixth day).

Consultation with the responsible cardiologist should, however, be done wherever necessary (e.g., in patients who have had recent percutaenous cardiac interventions [PCI]). Coronary artery stenting is used increasingly as a treatment for coronary artery disease. A period of anti platelet therapy is mandatory following coronary stenting, in order to minimize the risk of stent thrombosis. Approximately 5% of patients who undergo coronary stenting will require noncardiac surgery within 12 months, and the management of antiplatelet therapy in this setting is complex, requiring a balance between the risks of both operative haemorrhage and stent thrombosis.

High-risk patients proposed for "high-risk surgery" with an increased risk of bleeding should not be treated as outpatients.

Elderly patients with or without co-morbidity should be evaluated in accordance with accepted guidelines. It is useful if an elderly patent can be seen in advance of the procedure in order to make the necessary preparations. Minor perioperative cardiovascular events are not seen infrequently in the elderly. Preoperative ECG is of value as a base line and in order to exclude pre-existing severe arrhythmias or signs of ischemia.

Elderly patients may benefit from having their procedure performed without hospitalization so as to return to the home environment right after recovery. However, it is important to make adequate preparations and provide information not only to the patient but also to relatives/carers. It is also often of great help if the responsible GP is informed in order to be able to help and support the patient during the early postoperative stage if needed.

Obese patients and patients with history of any kind of sleep-related hypoventilation should be identified. Obesity is commonly associated with co-morbidity; diabetes, hypertension, ischemic heart disease, and obesity associated hypoventilation syndrome. All co-morbidities should be evaluated and controlled in accordance with set routines and it may emerge that in-hospital multi-disciplinary management is preferred for safety reasons.

Both obstructive sleep apnoea and the obesity hypoventilation syndrome result in physiological derangements that increase perioperative risk. Obesity is commonly associated with some degree of airway compromise during sleep, sedation, and post-anaesthesia. Obese patients have an increased risk of respiratory events during and in the postoperative period.

Smoking habits and any degree of sleep-associated breathing abnormality, sleep apnoea or related symptoms should be evaluated in the general patient population (see also the section on PONV).

3.1.4 **Diabetes**

Surgical stress often produces hyperglycemia in the perioperative period. Hyperglycemia has been shown to cause a significant increase in perioperative morbidity and mortality. It is the general consensus that strict glycaemic control is beneficial and should be achieved for diabetic patients in the perioperative period.

There is good evidence to show that controlling the blood glucose to < or = 10 mmol/l in the perioperative period for both types of diabetic patients improves outcome. The basic principle is as for in-hospital procedures that blood sugar control should be achieved with a glucose-insulin-potassium regimen in all type 1 diabetics and in type 2 diabetics undergoing moderate surgery.

Table 3.4 Glucose, Potassium, Insulin (GKI) or Alberti regimen

Blood glucose (mmol/l)	Soluble insulin (U) to be added to each 500 ml bag 5% glucose	Blood potassium (mmol/l)	KCl (mmol) to be added to each 500 ml bag 5% glucose
<4	5	<3	20
4–6	10	3–5	10
6.1–10	15	>5	None
10.1–20	20		
>20	Review	If potassium level not available, add 10 mmol KCl to each bag	

Table 3.4 is reproduced from *Oxford Handbook of Anaesthesia, Second Edition*, edited by Keith G. Allman and Iain H. Wilson, (2006), with permission from Oxford University Press

Patients with diabetes should be handled on an individual basis. Strict blood glucose control is recommended. Well-controlled patients on fast-acting insulin may follow a modified approach; Natof first described the principle as 'moving the sun in the sky'. In essence, this involves omitting the patient's breakfast and morning insulin, performing surgery first on the operating list, and subsequently resuming the patient's normal regimen as soon as possible after surgery, starting with the patient's usual morning insulin and breakfast.

Blood glucose concentrations should, regardless of which technique used, be carefully monitored during the perioperative period, aiming for a range of 5–13 mmol/l.

Intravenous glucose, potassium, insulin (GKI) in accordance with hospital guidelines is always an alternative for less well-controlled patients. Patients showing bad control (HbA1c > 8) should be referred for specialist consultation prior to surgery.

3.2 **Preoperative tests and investigations**

In minor surgery in the ASA scale 1–2 patient, preoperative tests are needed infrequently. In more extensive surgery and in patients with a medical history, laboratory testing, ECG, and eventually chest x-ray should be performed on an individual basis. Examples of surgical grades 1–4 are provided in Table 3.5. Preoperative tests by surgical grade and age are shown in Table 3.6.

Table 3.5 Examples of surgical grades

Surgical grades	Examples
Grade 1 (minor)	Excision skin lesion; drain breast abscess
Grade 2 (intermediate)	Inguinal hernia; varicose vein(s); tonsillectomy; arthroscopy
Grade 3 (major)	Hysterectomy; TURP; lumbar discectomy; thyroidectomy
Grade 4 (major +)	Joint replacement; thoracic operations; colonic resection; radical neck dissection

Table 3.5 is reproduced from *Oxford Handbook of Anaesthesia, Second Edition*, edited by Keith G. Allman and Iain H. Wilson, (2006), with permission from Oxford University Press.

Table 3.6 Preoperative tests by surgical grade and age

Surgra	Age	CXR	ECG	FBC	INR	U&E	Ranglu	Uri	Total
1	<16	NO	NO	NO	NO	NO	NO	NO	0
1	16–60	NO	NO	NO	NO	NO	NO	NO	0
1	61–80	NO	NO	NO	NO	NO	NO	NO	0
1	>80	NO	YES	NO	NO	NO	NO	NO	1
2	<16	NO	NO	NO	NO	NO	NO	NO	0
2	16–60	NO	NO	NO	NO	NO	NO	NO	0
2	61–80	NO	NO	YES	NO	NO	NO	NO	1
2	>80	NO	YES	YES	NO	NO	NO	NO	2
3	<16	NO	NO	NO	NO	NO	NO	NO	0
3	16–60	NO	NO	YES	NO	NO	NO	NO	1
3	61–80	NO	YES	YES	NO	YES	NO	NO	3
3	>80	NO	YES	YES	NO	YES	NO	NO	3
4	<16	NO	NO	NO	NO	NO	NO	NO	0
4	16–60	NO	NO	YES	NO	YES	NO	NO	2
4	61–80	NO	YES	YES	NO	YES	NO	NO	3
4	>80	NO	YES	YES	NO	YES	NO	NO	3

Notes: CXR = Chest X-ray. ECG = Electrocardiogram, FBC = Full blood count, INR = International normalized ratio, U&E = Urea and electrolytes, Ranglu = Random glucose, Uri = Urine.

Table 3.6 is reproduced from *Oxford Handbook of Anaesthesia, Second Edition*, edited by Keith G. Allman and Iain H. Wilson, (2006), with permission from Oxford University Press.

> **Box 3.1 Summary tips for setting up a day case anaesthesia service: patient selection and preparation**
>
> **Special demands**
>
> Yes—safe discharge within hours.
>
> **Converting from an in-hospital to a day case programme**
>
> Yes—proper selection and diversion—patients and procedures where safe discharge within hours can be ascertained.
>
> **Setting up a hospital based freestanding day case service**
>
> Safe discharge within hours is fundamental. Start with simple cases and procedures and expand successively based on experience.
>
> **Think about**
>
> Put patient safety first; if safety can be secured, plan for how to increase patient turnover and how to take on more complex procedures. Safety and quality of care should be followed continuously.

Further reading

Anaesthesia for the Elderly Edited by Chris Dodds, Chandra M. Kumar & Frederique Servin Oxford Anaesthesia Library.

Anaesthesia for the Overweight and Obese Patient Edited by Mark Bellamy & Michel Struys. Oxford Anaesthesia Library.

Berg C, Berger DH, Makia A, Whalen C, Albo D, Bellows C, Awad SS. Perioperative beta-blocker therapy and heart rate control during noncardiac surgery. *Am J Surg* 2007 Aug; **194**(2): 189-91.

Bergman SA. Perioperative management of the diabetic patient. *Oral Surg Oral Med Oral Pathol Oral Radiol Endod.* 2007 Jun; **103**(6): 731-7.

Cahill RA, McGreal GT, Crowe BH, Ryan DA, Manning BJ, Cahill MR, Redmond HP. Duration of increased bleeding tendency after cessation of aspirin therapy. *J Am Coll Surg.* 2005 Apr; **200**(4): 564-73.

Gregory L. Bryson *et al.* Patient selection in ambulatory anesthesia—An evidence-based review: part I. *Canadian J Anaesth* 2004; **51**(8): 768-81.

Jackson I, Smith I, Watson B. Peri-operative management of diabetes. *Anaesthesia.* 2007 Jun; **62**(6): 631-2.

Kaafarani HM, Atluri PV, Thornby J, Itani KM. Beta-blockade in noncardiac surgery: outcome at all levels of cardiac risk. *Arch Surg* 2008 Oct; **143**(10): 940-4.

Luckie MJ, Khattar RS, Fraser DG. Noncardiac Surgery and Antiplatelet Therapy Following Coronary Artery Stenting. *Heart.* 2009 Feb 12. E-publication ahead of printing.

Rehman HU, Mohammed K. Perioperative management of diabetic patients. *Curr Surg* 2003 Nov–Dec; **60**(6): 607–11. Review.

Robertshaw HJ, Hall GM. Diabetes mellitus: anaesthetic management. *Anaesthesia* 2006 Dec; **61**(12): 1187–90.

Rosenman DJ, McDonald FS, Ebbert JO, Erwin PJ, LaBella M, Montori VM. Clinical consequences of withholding versus administering renin-angiotensin-aldosterone system antagonists in the preoperative period. *J Hosp Med* 2008 Jul; **3**(4): 319–25.

Servin F. Low-dose aspirin and clopidogrel: how to act in patients scheduled for day surgery. *Curr Opin Anaesthesiol* 2007 Dec; **20**(6): 531–4. Review.

Shnaider I, Chung F. Outcomes in day surgery. *Curr Opin Anaesthesiol.* 2006 Dec; **19**(6): 622–9.

Chapter 4

Analgesics in day case surgery

Key points

- The day case patient is to leave the hospital within hours following surgery; thus special emphasis must be placed on providing adequate pain management throughout the perioperative course as well as following discharge.
- Information and active coaching of the patient through the entire perioperative period is of great importance; patient satisfaction is important and efforts should be focused on obtaining adequate pain relief with minimum side effects.
- A multi-modal pain management strategy has become the gold standard. Pain management should already have been addressed in preoperative preparation and information. Provide the patient with a prescription in order to have adequate medication at home after return from the procedure or provide take-home medications and information about their use.
- The use of local anaesthesia intraoperatively, fast-acting anaesthesia prior to incision and long-acting anaesthesia at skin closure, should be advocated strongly wherever possible; this pre-incision and at-wound-closure technique should also be used in patients who undergo surgery under general anaesthesia, as it helps to reduce the noxious influx and thus reduce the pain intra as well as postoperatively.
- Intraoperative opioid analgesics should be used where needed but at the lowest effective dose.
- Postoperative pain management is based on a long acting local anaesthetic in the wound at closure, and oral pain medications (NSAID or "coxib" for 3–5–7 days and additional paracetamol 1 g up to four times daily) and further availability of an oral opioid as a rescue pain medication when needed.
- For more painful procedures, a long-acting slow-release oral opioid should be added and a fast-acting oral opioid provided as rescue pain therapy in order to handle incidences of "breakthrough" pain.

Securing adequate pain management is one of the major goals in day surgical anaesthesia. **Patients should be ready for safe discharge within hours whilst still maintaining quality of care, provided that there is adequate pain therapy**. The overall pain management achieved is therefore of utmost importance. The pain therapy pyramid is shown in Figure 4.1.

4.1 Balanced analgesia or multi-modal analgesia

Multi-modal analgesia has become the "gold standard" in day case anaesthesia. Combining drugs with different modes of action, thereby creating additive or synergistic analgesic effects and minimizing the occurrence and extent of side effects, is one of the most important aspects of day case anaesthesia. A simple pain management pyramid is shown in Figure 4.1.

4.1.1 Local anaesthesia is one part of multi-modal analgesia

Local anaesthesia has a long history of use in superficial minor office-based surgery. The modern amide local anaesthetics are associated with low toxicity and their use is strongly recommended whenever possible.

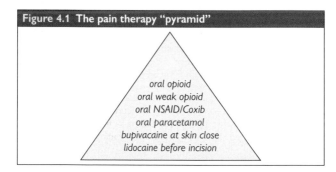

Figure 4.1 The pain therapy "pyramid"

oral opioid
oral weak opioid
oral NSAID/Coxib
oral paracetamol
bupivacaine at skin close
lidocaine before incision

Infiltration of the wound and/or nerve block before surgery, prior to incision, is strongly recommended. Surgical incisions should not be made without blocking the nociceptive inflow to the spinal cord regardless of whether the patient is scheduled to undergo general anaesthesia, sedation or to be fully awake during the procedure in order to minimize the stress response. Administration of fast-acting local anaesthesia prior to incision followed by the provision of long-acting local anaesthesia at wound closure should be regarded as a basic routine. Local anaesthesia is a simple, safe, and effective way to reduce noxious inflow as well as the need for other analgesics/anaesthetics during and after surgery.

The route of administration may vary from simple wound infiltration, to infiltration of troachar ports, to injection into the joint to perform various forms of nerve blocks.

Single infiltration or block is helpful both during and after surgery, reducing the need for opioid analgesia and thereby reducing opioid-associated side-effects intraoperatively as well as postoperatively.

4.2 **Regional anaesthesia: perineural blocks**

The vast majority of nerves can be blocked effectively. Performing a nerve block is a matter of skill and experience. Proper training is fundamental in order to achieve acceptable success rates. A properly performed single-injection block provides surgical anaesthesia and, when higher concentrations of local anaesthesia solutions have been used, also muscle relaxation. There are also various options for catheter techniques. Catheters may be placed either in the wound area or the para-neuronal area in order to provide a sensory block. Both continuous local anaesthesia and intermittent bolus techniques can be used with impressive effects on postoperative pain in intermediate/major surgery. The catheter technique has been shown to be most effective in reducing pain, for instance in hand and shoulder surgery.

Peripheral blocks can either be performed alone or in combination with wound infiltration. The maximum dose in order to avoid any risk of system toxicity must of course be kept in mind. Effective block of the noxious inflow from the surgical site dramatically decreases the need for intraoperative analgesia, and anaesthesia can be kept to a minimal level.

Detailed recommendations regarding techniques and proper procedures for performing peripheral nerve blocks is outside of the scope of this pocketbook; however several textbooks, full-colour picture atlases, and interactive DVDs are currently available which detail how to best perform peripheral blocks. A few of these publications have been listed along with the further reading list at the end of this chapter.

Ultrasound guidance for regional blocks has become an increasingly popular technique, and a recent meta-analysis published by Abrahams in the *British Journal of Anaesthesia* has documented its superiority in achieving successful blocks. A number of books have recently been published on the use of the ultrasound guidance technique for regional blocks and a few of these are also listed and the end of this chapter.

The perineural techniques offer interesting and important benefits, but the risks versus benefits must be acknowledged and skill in the performance of these techniques should be ascertained. General recommendations and guidelines are currently under development in many countries in order to encourage and ascertain good clinical practice. The National Institute for Health in the UK has recently issued a guideline document regarding the safe use of this technique (see http://www.nice.org.uk/nicemedia/pdf/IPG285Guidance.pdf). Common techniques of regional anaesthesia used in orthopaedics are listed in Tables 4.1–4.4.

Table 4.1 Plexus blocks of the upper extremities		
Technique	**Neural Target/ Indications**	**Comments**
Interscalene block	Target: Root-to-trunk transition (interscalene space). Indications: Proximal procedures of arm; requires supplementation with ulnar nerve block for procedures of forearm and hand.	Injection Volume: 10–15 ml (ultrasound); otherwise, 20–40 ml.
Supraclavicular block	Target: Trunk-to-division transition. Indications: Procedures of the arm, elbow, or forearm.	Injection Volume: 10–15 ml (ultrasound highly desirable; if unavailable, use infraclavicular block).
Infraclavicular block	Target: Posterior, lateral, and medial cords. Indications: Procedures of the elbow, forearm, and hand.	Injection Volume: 7–11 ml per neural cord (ultrasound); otherwise, one 20–30 ml) injection. Compared with axillary block, has advantage of not requiring supplemental injection of musculocutaneous nerve. If ultrasound and nerve stimulation are unavailable unavailable, forego above advantage, and use axillary block.

Table 4.1 (Contd.)

Technique	Neural Target/ Indications	Comments
Axillary block	Target: Radial, ulnar, and median nerves. Indications: Procedures of elbow, forearm, and hand.	Injection Volume: 5–8 ml per nerve (ultrasound). If ultrasound is unavailable, several options still exist: 35–40 ml (single injection); 10 ml (near each of the three nerves); two 20 ml injections (transarterial approach); or 40–50 ml (fascial click method). Compared with infraclavicular block, can be performed in the absence of ultrasound or nerve stimulation. Requires supplemental injection of musculocutaneous nerve

Table 4.1 is reproduced with permission from Latifzai *et al.* (2008) Orthopaedic anaesthesia Part 2. Common techniques of regional anaesthesia in orthopaedics. *Bulletin of the NYU Hospital for Joint Diseases* **66**(4): 306–16.

Table 4.2 Peripheral blocks at the elbow, wrist, and digits

Technique	Neural Target/ Indications	Comments
Elbow block	Target: Median, radial, musculocutaneous, and ulnar nerves. Indications: Procedures of the hand.	Injection Volume: 3–5 ml per each nerve.
Wrist block	Target: Median, radial, and ulnar nerves. Indications: General or site-specific procedures of the hand.	Injection Volume: 3–5 ml (median nerve), a total of 6–8 ml (radial nerve), 4–8 ml (ulnar nerve).
Digital block	Target: The four digital nerves. Indications: Minor procedures of the fingers.	Injection Volume: 1–2 ml (per each of the four nerves using the ring approach); 2 ml (per each of the two sides using the transthecal approach). Using epinephrine must be avoided.

Table 4.2 is reproduced with permission from Latifzai *et al.* (2008) Orthopaedic anaesthesia Part 2. Common techniques of regional anaesthesia in orthopaedics. *Bulletin of the NYU Hospital for Joint Diseases* **66**(4): 306–16.

Table 4.3 Plexus blocks of the lower extremities

Technique	Neural Target/ Indications	Comments
Femoral nerve block	Target: The femoral nerve. Indications: Operative procedures involving anterior thigh (e.g., quadriceps tendon, patella), perioperative analgesia (e.g., total knee arthroplasty, femoral shaft surgery).	Injection volume: 20 ml (ultrasound); otherwise, 20–30 ml.
3-in-1 block	Target: Femoral, obturator, and lateral cutaneous nerves. Indications: Same as those mentioned for femoral nerve block, However, has the added feature of being used in combination with sciatic nerve block for anaesthesia of entire limb (distal to mid-thigh).	Injection volume: 20 ml (ultrasound); otherwise 20–40 ml.
Saphenous nerve block	Target: Saphenous nerve. Indications: Procedures distal to the knee (when combined with sciatic nerve block), or distal to the ankle (when combined with popliteal block).	Injection volume: 5–10 ml around the saphenous vein (using ultrasound); or a similar volume using a ring approach.
Sciatic nerve block	Target: sciatic nerve. Indications: Can be combined with 3-in-1 block for procedures distal to the mid-thigh, or with femoral/ saphenous nerve blocks for procedures distal to the knee.	Injection volume: 20 ml (ultrasound) or 20–30 ml (without ultrasound) using the Labat technique. If using an anterior approach, 20–25 ml.

Table 4.3 is reproduced with permission from Latifzai et al. (2008) Orthopaedic anaesthesia Part 2. Common techniques of regional anaesthesia in orthopaedics. *Bulletin of the NYU Hospital for Joint Diseases* **66**(4): 306–16.

Table 4.4 Peripheral blocks at the popliteal fossa, ankle, and digits

Technique	Neural Target/ Indications	Comments
Popliteal block	Target: Sciatic nerve (prior to its division into the common peroneal and tibial nerves). Indications: Foot and ankle surgery (should be combined with saphenous block if medial aspect of foot involved).	Injection volume: 30 ml (ultrasound); otherwise. 10–30 ml.
Ankle block	Target: The posterior tibial, sural superficial and deep peroneal, and saphenous nerves. Indications: Procedures of the foot.	Injection volume 3–5 ml (paresthesia); otherwise, 7–10 ml for the posterior tibial nerve 3–5 ml for the deep peroneal nerve, and the saphenous nerve. 5–7 ml for the sural nerve, and the superficial peroneal nerve.
Digital block	Target: The four digital nerves. Indications: minor procedures of the toes.	Injection volume: 1–1.5 ml (per each of the four nerves of the great toe). 1.5 ml (per each of the two sides of the four lateral toes). Using epinephrine must be avoided.

Table 4.4 is reproduced with permission from Latifzai et al. (2008) Orthopaedic anaesthesia Part 2. Common techniques of regional anaesthesia in orthopaedics. *Bulletin of the NYU Hospital for Joint Diseases* **66**(4): 306–16.

31

The simple peripheral blocks and simple wound infiltration should not be forgotten. A simple digital nerve block, such as a classical four-point digital nerve block, is a simple, safe and easy-to-perform technique for distal extremity surgery. An ankle block is a safe technique that is easily learned and renders a high success rate also without sophisticated technical support. The basics for successful performance of the, e.g., ankle block are the use of a fast-acting amide local anaesthetic (e.g., lidocaine 10 mg/ml) in rather huge volumes.

4.2.1 Which local anaesthetic?

The choice of local anaesthetic drug used for day case surgical procedures is of great importance. A list of local anaesthetic agents commonly used for day surgery is listed in Box 4.1.

All the fast-acting local anaesthetics (e.g., lidocaine, mepivacaine, or prilocaine) can be used for infiltration or provision of peripheral blocks. A solution with 10 mg/ml is sufficient to provide adequate intraoperative anaesthesia. The three amide local anaesthetics mentioned provide rapid onset within 3 to 10 minutes.

Lidocaine, mepivacaine and prilocaine have a moderate duration of action (1–2 hr). Bupivacaine, levobupivacaine, or ropivacaine have a somewhat slower onset, but give long-lasting local anaesthesia; pain relief is commonly achieved for up to 6 to 10 hours. A summary of clinical characteristics of different local anaesthetic agents is shown in Table 4.5.

For each individual agent, the duration of analgesia will be determined by the agent used, the addition of vasoconstriction, and the total dose of the drug administered. High concentration and small volume will increase the "depth" of the block, but will limit the extension, whist a low concentration will reduce the number of nerve "fibres" blocked. The volume will have major impact of the area anaesthetized.

Box 4.1 Local anaesthetic drugs commonly used in day case anaesthesia

Fast acting/short duration
- Lidocaine
- Mepivacaine
- Prilocaine

Long acting
- Bupivacaine
- Levobupivacaine
- Ropivacaine

Table 4.5 Characteristics of different local anaesthetic agents						
Agent	pKa	Relative lipid solubility	Relative potency	Protein binding (%)	Onset	Duration
Procaine	8.9	1	1	6	Slow	Short
Amethocaine	8.5	200	8	75	Slow	Long
Lidocaine	7.7	150	2	65	Fast	Medium
Prilocaine	7.7	50	2	55	Fast	Medium
Etidocaine	7.7	5000	6	96	Fast	Long
Mepivacaine	7.6	50	2	78	Fast	Medium
Ropivacaine	8.1	400	6	94	Med	Long
Bupivacaine	8.1	1000	8	95	Med	Long
Levobupivacaine	8.1	1000	8	95	Med	Long

Table 4.5 is reproduced from *Oxford Handbook of Anaesthesia, Second Edition*, edited by Keith G. Allman and Iain H. Wilson, (2006), with permission from Oxford University Press.

The effect of vasoconstrictors may be preferred in order to reduce perioperative bleeding and to prolong the duration of anaesthesia. The effect on duration, however, depends on the local anaesthetic used and the site of the injection. Adding a vasoconstrictor will prolong the action for the short-acting agents from 50% to 100%. The prolongation of analgesia duration is less for the long-acting agents. The addition of adrenaline reduces the peak concentration in the blood for short-acting as well as long-acting local anaesthetics and thus also the risk for systemic toxicity, but the degree of this reduction depends on the site of injection and the specific local anaesthetic agent injected.

General dose recommendations for local anaesthetics commonly used in day case anaesthesia are provided in Table 4.6.

Combining local anaesthesia with morphine and other adjuncts has been used for prolongation of anaesthesia, especially intra-articular local anaesthesia, for a long time. Analgesia from single injection local anaesthesia intra-articular after arthroscopy may be prolonged by adding morphine and ketorolac. One regimen shown to be effective for intra-articular injection for post-operative pain relief is ropivacaine 150 mg, morphine 4 mg, and ketorolac 30 mg mixed with saline to a total volume of 30 ml. Patients administered the triple mixture required less oral analgeiscs on day 1 (P<.05), had less sleep disturbances because of pain, more patients were ready to work on days 1 and 2 (P<.05), and were more satisfied on days 1 and 4 to 7 than patients administered with ropivacaine only.

4.2.2 Toxicity of local anaesthesia

Local anaesthetic agents are relatively free from side effects if they are administered in appropriate doses and in the correct anatomical location. However, systemic toxic reactions may occur, usually as a result of accidental intravascular administration or excessive doses. Systemic reactions to local anaesthetics are primarily associated with central nervous system (CNS) and the cardiovascular system. Early signs are nausea, hypotension, dizziness, paresthesias and confusion. A summary of clinical profiles of different uses of local anaesthesia is shown in Table 4.7.

Prilocaine may cause increase in methaemoglobin and it should be used with caution in higher doses in patients with a critical oxygen saturation or oxygen delivery.

Table 4.6 General dose recommendations for local anaesthetics commonly used in day case surgery

Agent	Maximum recommended doses	Maximum recommended doses with vasoconstrictor
Bupivacaine	2 mg/kg	2 mg/kg
Levobupivacaine	2 mg/kg	2 mg/kg
Ropivacaine	3 mg/kg	3 mg/kg
Lidocaine	3 mg/kg	6 mg/kg
Prilocaine	6 mg/kg	8 mg/kg
Cocaine	1.5-3 mg/kg	

Table 4.6 is reproduced from *Oxford Handbook of Anaesthesia, Second Edition*, edited by Keith G. Allman and Iain H. Wilson, (2006), with permission from Oxford University Press.

Table 4.7 Clinical profiles of different uses of local anaesthesia

	Surgical site infiltration	Peripheral nerve block	Regional blocks
Easy to perform	+++	++	+
Selectivity	+++	++	+
Complication/risk	Low	Low	Low/intermediate

4.3 Intraoperative opioids

The profound synergistic effect between opioids and inhaled anaesthetics as well as propofol is well recognized. The use of small opiate doses drastically reduces the need for main anaesthetics such as propofol as well as halogenated anaesthetics (see also chapter 5 on anaesthetics in day surgery).

The choice of intraoperative opioid is a matter of personal choice. Small doses of fentanyl, alfentanil, or a continuous infusion of remifentanil are all suitable alternatives. However, every attempt should be made to minimize the need for and use of opioids throughout the perioperative period. If adequate analgesia and stress response can be achieved with local anaesthesia and/or other non-opioid analgesics, the intraoperative use of any opioid should be avoided.

Figures 4.2 and 4.3 show drug interactions between commonly used anaesthetics and analgesics.

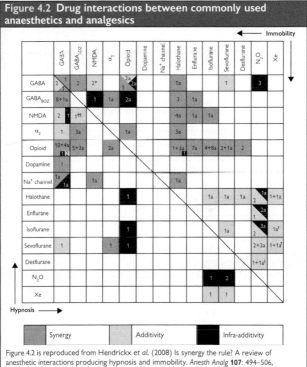

Figure 4.2 Drug interactions between commonly used anaesthetics and analgesics

Figure 4.2 is reproduced from Hendrickx et al. (2008) Is synergy the rule? A review of anesthetic interactions producing hypnosis and immobility. *Anesth Analg* **107**: 494–506, © Lippincott, Williams & Wilkins.

35

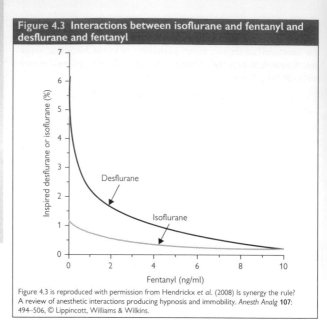

Figure 4.3 Interactions between isoflurane and fentanyl and desflurane and fentanyl

Figure 4.3 is reproduced with permission from Hendrickx et al. (2008) Is synergy the rule? A review of anesthetic interactions producing hypnosis and immobility. *Anesth Analg* **107**: 494–506, © Lippincott, Williams & Wilkins.

4.4 Postoperative pain management

In day case/office-based surgery, providing full preoperative information (both oral and written) regarding the postoperative pain management strategy is of outmost importance. The team must ensure that the patient understands the extent of the surgical procedure and the postoperative course, and that the patient is capable of coping with recovery in the home environment.

A motivated and well-informed patient who is aware of the pain pattern, rehabilitation scheme and pain medication strategy is much better off than a less well-informed patient. Patients' expectations have an important impact on their overall satisfaction.

Patients should be informed about early mobilization and discharge and should be warned not to expect a protracted bed rest in hospital following the procedure. Procedure-specific pain medication schemes should be available based on multi-modal pain management.

Patients must be informed preoperatively about the need for adequate transport back home; the availability of a person to take the patient home following the procedure is of huge value and is strongly recommended. Going home in a taxi without an accompanying person may be appropriate following procedures performed under local anaesthesia or in combination with light sedation only. However, patients who have received general anaesthesia may get nauseated or may start to feel fatigue. Putting a patient who has been under general anaesthesia in a taxi without company following surgery is risky, both for the patient and the taxi driver.

4.4.1 Local anaesthesia (single shot or continuous catheter technique)

The basic concept of using a fast-acting anaesthetic agent prior to incision and wound infiltration with a long-acting local anaesthetic during or right after wound closure is of great value in order to reduce the early experience of postoperative pain and thereby to facilitate mobilization and discharge.

Oral paracetamol, non-steroidal anti-inflammatory drugs (NSAIDs)/ "coxibs", weak opioids and, when needed, strong opioids are the basis of the postoperative pain management strategy in most day case surgical procedures. Continuous local anaesthesia infusion from a paraneural or wound catheter 'home pump delivery system' may be an option (see also section 4.4.8).

4.4.2 Paracetamol

The basic medication consists of paracetamol 1 g up to four times daily. Oral administration is preferred. The effervescent preparation of paracetamol has been shown to create rapid and predictable plasma concentration within 20–40 minutes. Oral administration is preferred to rectal administration from a kinetic point of view.

Intravenous administration is an option during the intraoperative period if needed.

Box 4.2 shows the Cochrane analysis regarding the use of oral paracetamol (acetaminophen) for postoperative pain relief in adults.

Much of the effect of paracetamol involves central mechanisms involving serotonergic receptors. Paracetamol is most likely a central analgesic drug that must be distinguished from NSAIDs, which justifies the usual combination of paracetamol in postoperative pain.

Box 4.2 Cochrane analysis of the use of oral paracetamol for postoperative pain relief

"This review assessed data from fifty-one studies and found that paracetamol provided effective pain relief for about half of participants experiencing moderate to severe pain after an operation, including dental surgery for a period of about four hours. There were no clear differences between doses of paracetamol typically used. These single dose studies did not associate paracetamol with any serious side effects."

The mechanism of action raises the potential for a negative interaction between paracetamol and 5-HT3-receptor antagonists. Some studies suggest that the co-administration of tropisetron or granisetron with paracetamol can potentially block the analgesic effect of paracetamol. These effects have however not been confirmed or disproved by clinical studies.

4.4.3 NSAIDs/COX-II inhibitors

Non-steroidal anti-inflammatory drugs (NSAIDs) bind to and block the cycloxygenase receptor and thus inhibit the production of prostaglandins. The more selective blockers of cycloxygenase II or inducible cycloxygenase were introduced in order to lower the incidence and severity of gastrointestinal side effects seen with the non-selective NSAIDs. Today both non-selective NSAIDs and selective COX-II inhibitors (so-called "Coxibs") are available.

The oral route is effective and is the preferred route of administration of NSAIDs/COX-II inhibitors.

The risks for gastrointestinal side effects when used for longer periods of time should be acknowledged, and in patients with history of severe gastritis and/or gastric ulcer, the risk versus benefit should be carefully evaluated.

Both Coxibs and traditional NSAIDs should also be avoided in patients with any signs or history of unstable cardiovascular disease. The potential risk for cardiovascular events that has been associated with the use of Coxibs and NSAIDs should be kept in mind.

One should also be aware that there is experimental data showing that NSAIDs/Coxibs may influence the healing process. The clinical relevance of the effects on the healing process and bone repair is still a matter of debate. In patients with other factors impairing bone healing, such as heavy smoking, bad circulation and osteoporosis, the risks versus benefits must of course be considered.

When used short term at the lowest effective dose, however, NSAIDs/Coxibs provide analgesia seemingly without significant toxicity.

Although non-specific NSAIDs provides similar analgesia to Coxibs, the use of non-specific NSAIDs has been somewhat limited in the perioperative setting because of their "side effects", their effects on platelet function potentially increasing the risk for bleeding and haematoma.

Coxibs may be a safer alternative in that setting, as they do not lead to coagulation dysfunction and no increased risk of bleeding/blood loss, which has been documented also in major orthopaedic cases.

The analgesic potency has been documented repeatedly and, in the meta-analysis of oral analgesics, the number needed to treat (NNT) is by far lowest for the Coxib group.

Figure 4.4 shows how to build a stepwise postoperative pain management ladder.

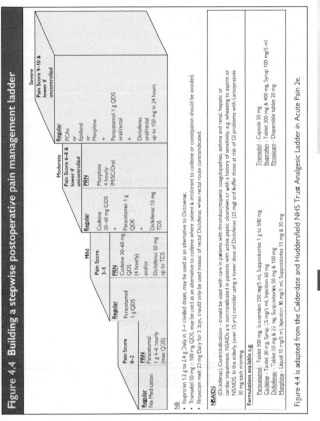

Figure 4.4 Building a stepwise postoperative pain management ladder

	Pain Score 0–2	Mild Pain Score 3–5	Moderate Pain Score 6–8 & lower if uncontrolled	Severe Pain Score 9–10 & lower if uncontrolled
Regular No Medication	**Regular** Paracetamol 1 g QDS	**Regular** Codeine 30–60 mg QDS + Paracetamol 1 g QDS + Diclofenac 50 mg TDS	**Regular** Morphine 4 hourly IM/SC/Oral	**Regular** PCAs or Epidural or Morphine + Paracetamol 1 g QDS oral/rectal + Diclofenac oral/rectal up to 150 mg in 24 hours
	PRN Paracetamol 1 g 4–6 hourly (max QDS)	**PRN** Codeine 30–60 mg QDS (4 hourly) and/or Diclofenac 50 mg up to TDS	**PRN** Morphine 4 hourly IM/SC/Oral	

NB

- Ibuprofen 1.2 g to 2.4 g Daily in 3–4 divided doses, may be used as an alternative to Diclofenac.
- Tramadol 50 mg – 100 mg QDS, may be used as an alternative to codeine where patient is intolerant to codeine or constipation should be avoided.
- Piroxicam melt 20 mg Daily for 3 days, should only be used instead of rectal Diclofenac when rectal route contraindicated.

NSAIDs

(Diclofenac) Contraindications - should be used with care in patients with thrombocytopenic coagulopathies, asthma and renal, hepatic or cardiac impairment. NSAIDs are contraindicated in patients with active peptic ulceration or with a history of sensitivity, e.g. wheezing to aspirin or NSAIDS. In the elderly (over 75 yrs) consider using a lower dose of Diclofenac (25 mg) and buffer those at risk of GI problems with Lansoprazole 30 mg each morning.

Formulations available e.g.

Paracetamol - Tablet 500 mg, Suspension 250 mg/5 ml, Suppositories 1 g to 500 mg
Codeine - Tablet 30 mg, Syrup 25 mg/5 ml, Injection 60 mg
Diclofenac - Tablet 50 mg & 25 mg, Suppositories 50 mg & 100 mg
Morphine - Liquid 10 mg/5 ml, Injection 10 mg/1 ml, Suppositories 15 mg & 30 mg

Tramadol - Capsule 50 mg
Ibuprofen - Tablet 200 mg & 400 mg, Syrup 100 mg/5 ml
Piroxicam - Dispersible tablet 20 mg

Figure 4.4 is adapted from the Calderdale and Huddersfield NHS Trust Analgesic Ladder in Acute Pain 2e.

4.4.3.1 *Traditional NSAIDs: simple, safe and well-established*

Diclofenac is an NSAID with a long history in clinical practice. It is one of the classic NSAID drugs that have pain-relieving properties. Diclofenac is used to treat many conditions, one of which is acute postoperative pain. Box 4.3 summarizes the findings of the latest Cochrane review regarding the use of diclofenac.

4.4.3.2 *Coxibs: development with some benefits*

Celecoxib was one of the first of the new-generation of NSAIDs known as COX-II inhibitors. Compared with conventional NSAIDs, celecoxib has fewer gastrointestinal side effects with long-term use. Celecoxib is used for the relief of chronic pain caused by osteoarthritis and rheumatoid arthritis. It also has gained increasing interest for the management of postoperative pain. Box 4.4 summarizes the most recent Cochrane analysis regarding the use of celecoxib.

Several studies have shown coxibs to reduce the need for opioid analgesics and improve the recovery process. Coxibs have been shown effective in reducing pain after general surgery, gynaecological surgery, as well as orthopaedic surgery. When initiated already prior to surgery favourable effects on intra and postoperative pain has been shown without any signs of adverse effects.

> **Box 4.3 Cochrane analysis of the use of diclofenac for postoperative pain relief**
>
> "A single dose oral diclofenac provides effective pain relief for adults experiencing moderate or severe pain following a surgical procedure. There was no significant difference between diclofenac sodium and diclofenac potassium although there were few data for this analysis. The incidence of adverse effects did not differ significantly from placebo."

> **Box 4.4 Cochrane analysis of the use of celecoxib for postoperative pain relief**
>
> "This review examined the efficacy of celecoxib in relieving acute pain. Eight trials provided data. A 200 mg dose of celecoxib was at least as effective as aspirin 600/650 mg and paracetamol (acetaminophen) 1000 mg for relieving postoperative pain, while a 400 mg dose was at least as effective as ibuprofen 400 mg. Adverse events occurred at a similar rate with celecoxib and placebo. One serious adverse event (rhabdomyolysis—muscle breakdown) was probably related to celecoxib. Withdrawals due to adverse events were few and occurred at similar rates with celecoxib and placebo."

4.4.4 **Weak opioids**

The next step in postoperative pain management is to add a weak opioid. A weak opioid should also be the alternative when NSAIDs/Coxibs are contraindicated.

Dihydrocodeine treatment of acute postoperative pain has been evaluated in a Cochrane review. This review assessed the efficacy of single-dose dihydrocodeine in adults with moderate/severe postoperative pain using information from randomized placebo controlled trials (see Box 4.5).

Dextropropoxyphene administered in a single dose taken on its own and also in combination with paracetamol to treat postoperative pain was evaluated in a recent Cochrane analysis. This review assessed the analgesic efficacy and adverse effects that single dose oral dextropropoxyphene taken alone or in combination with paracetamol had in treating moderate to severe postoperative pain (see Box 4.6).

Tramadol has also been used extensively for pain management in day case surgery. Tramadol has a dual mechanism of action: weak mu-opioid-receptor agonist and a reuptake inhibitor of serotonin and noradrenaline, whereas oxycodone is a traditional opioid analgesic. Meta-analysis has shown that tramadol or tramadol/paracetamol in combination decreases pain intensity, produces symptom relief, and improves function, but these benefits are rather limited. Adverse events, although reversible and not life threatening, often cause

> #### Box 4.5 **Cochrane analysis of the use of dihydrocodeine for postoperative pain relief**
>
> "There was a lack of data that could be included in the analyses; all assessed the oral form of the drug and none assessed dihydrocodeine 60 mg. The results were not robust. The implication was that single-dose oral dihydrocodeine 30 mg was more effective than placebo, but was inferior to ibuprofen 400 mg. Dizziness, drowsiness and confusion were commonly reported."

> #### Box 4.6 **Cochrane analysis of the use of dextropropoxyphene for postoperative pain relief**
>
> "The combination of dextropropoxyphene 65 mg with paracetamol 650 mg showed similar efficacy to that of tramadol 100 mg for single dose studies in postoperative pain but with a lower incidence of side effects. This review also highlighted that Ibuprofen 400 mg was yet more effective than both tramadol 100 mg and dextropropoxyphene 650 mg."

participants to stop taking the medication and could limit the usefulness of tramadol or tramadol plus paracetamol.

4.4.5 Opioids

Modified release Slow-release oxycodone orally has been found to be safe and effective in day surgery, it is recommended that patients receive tablets of m/r oxycodone to be taken twice daily as a supplement to the base-line NSAID/Coxib/paracetamol regimen.

A Cochrane analysis has evaluated the effects of oxycodone. This review assessed the efficacy of single-dose oral oxycodone and oxycodone plus paracetamol in adults with moderate/severe postoperative pain using information from randomized placebo-controlled trials (see Box 4.7).

M/r oxycodone 10 mg orally twice daily in combination with paracetamol is a reasonable alternative for patients who should not be prescribed NSAIDs/Coxibs.

Tramadol and paracetamol in combination may also be an option in patients who should not receive NSAIDs/Coxibs.

A good analgesic protocol which provides adequate pain relief and which is easy to follow—thereby assuring a high patient compliance—in combination with minimum side effects such as tiredness, nausea, and vomiting, is of outmost importance in day surgery.

Postoperative pain management should begin either before or immediately after the end of surgery with an oral dose of, e.g., oral diclofenac 50 mg or etoricoxib 120 mg and a loading dose of 25–30 mg per kg of paracetamol orally.

There is increasing evidence for the benefits of preoperative NSAID/Coxib administration. Providing the patient with a preoperative Coxib has been shown to reduce postoperative pain and to reduce the need for rescue analgesia and also potentially reduce the need for intraoperative analgesia/anaesthesia. The number needed to treat league table is shown in Figure 4.5.

Box 4.7 Cochrane analysis of the use of oxycodone for postoperative pain relief

"The results were based on few data and were not robust. The implication was that these drugs were effective, providing similar analgesia to intramuscular morphine 10 mg and non-steroidal anti-inflammatory drugs. A dose-response relationship was not shown with increased doses of oxycodone or paracetamol. This may be due to the paucity of information. Drowsiness, dizziness, nausea and vomiting were commonly reported."

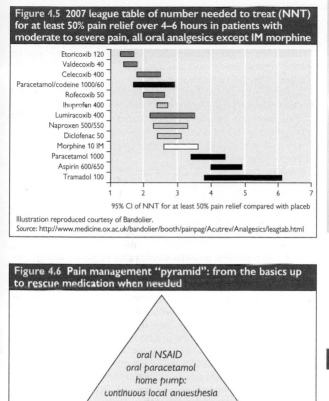

Figure 4.5 2007 league table of number needed to treat (NNT) for at least 50% pain relief over 4–6 hours in patients with moderate to severe pain, all oral analgesics except IM morphine

95% CI of NNT for at least 50% pain relief compared with placebo

Illustration reproduced courtesy of Bandolier.

Source: http://www.medicine.ox.ac.uk/bandolier/booth/painpag/Acutrev/Analgesics/leagtab.html

Figure 4.6 Pain management "pyramid": from the basics up to rescue medication when needed

oral NSAID
oral paracetamol
home pump:
continuous local anaesthesia

4.4.6 For how long should analgesics be prescribed?

Both pain intensity and duration of pain is individual. Postoperative pain management should therefore include not only a base medication/medications but analgesics to take when needed, as rescue medication. Analgesics should be available for at least up to a week. The patients should of course be informed to reduce taking analgesics as pain ceases. Similar to the stepwise addition of more potent analgesics, it is natural to reduce pain medication in a similar fashion. Paracetamol with its minimal number of side effects should be the last analgesic to be used when pain diminishes (up to 4g daily).

4.4.7 **Analgesics adjuncts**

The additional effect from other adjunct pain medications is not conclusive and different studies provide diverse results.

Gabapentin has been found to be effective in reducing the need for opioids in some studies, but the overall effect on pain and patients' satisfaction has still not been shown convincingly.

Clonidine in small doses may have a small opioid-sparing effect, but its exact role in clinical practice is still not clear.

Some protocols include low-dose ketamine. This is mostly seen intraoperatively in protocols where spontaneous breathing and free airway is of utmost importance to gain analgesia with a minimum of respiratory depression.

Providing thorough oral and written information regarding pain management is of great importance. Patients should be given explicit simple instructions on pain medication: which drugs, how often, and for how long. These instructions should also include explicit ways of acting in cases of inadequate pain control, what analgesics should be taken, and how frequently they can be used as rescue therapy.

4.4.8 **Postoperative patient-controlled regional analgesia (PCRA) at home**

Postoperative analgesia is generally limited to 12–16 h or less after a single-injection peripheral nerve block or local infiltration. Postoperative analgesia may be provided with a local anaesthetic infusion via a wound or perineural catheter after initial block resolution. This technique may now be used in the outpatient setting with the relatively recent introduction of reliable, portable infusion pumps. The technique using, e.g., an elastometric balloon pump, 'a home pump system' which allows the patient to self-administer local anaesthetic analgesia at home, has become an interesting and effective alternative in procedures with more extensive postoperative pain where good postoperative pain control may be hard to achieve with the basic combination of paracetamol/NSAID/weak opioid. The technique involves the placement of a multi-hole, thin (22-gauge) epidural or Perifix brachial plexus catheters (B. Braun, Melsungen, Germany) subcutaneously into the surgical wound, subacromially, intra-articularly, or in close proximity of a nerve or plexus. The catheter is tunnelled 4–5 cm subcutaneously by the surgeon and firmly secured on the skin by sterile tape. The catheter is placed and secured in position by the anaesthetist. The catheters are introduced 3–5 cm within the sheath and secured to the skin by transparent dressing and tape.

The elastomeric pump is available in a variety of models and volumes (http://www.iflo.com/).

An illustration of the elastometric ballon pump system is provided in Figure 4.7.

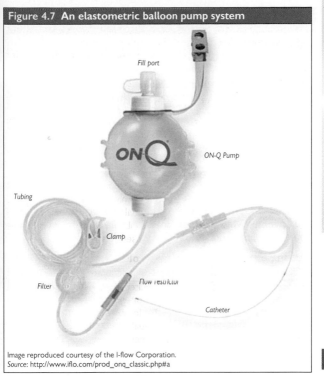

Figure 4.7 An elastometric balloon pump system

Fill port

ON-Q Pump

Tubing

Clamp

Filter

Flow restrictor

Catheter

Image reproduced courtesy of the I-flow Corporation.
Source: http://www.iflo.com/prod_onq_classic.php#a

The flow rate varies between 0.5 to 10 ml per hour with or without the option for patient bolus. Weak bupivacaine, levobupivacaine (1.25 mg/ml) or ropivacaine (2 mg/ml) is usually sufficient for adequate pain management.

Examples of protocols for managing post shoulder surgery are an interscalene catheter connected to an automated infusion pump delivering ropivacaine 0.2% (500 ml reservoir) with a basal rate of 8 ml/h and a 2 ml patient-controlled bolus available each hour. An alternative is using a patient-controlled interscalene analgesia with 0.125% levobupivacaine with a basal infusion rate, 6 ml/h; bolus, 2 ml; lockout period, 15 min; maximum three boluses per hour. Both have been shown to provide adequate pain relief and recovery of motor function after open shoulder surgery.

The pain management pyramid when a catheter is placed para-neural, intra-articular, or in the wound for local anaesthesia, is shown in Figure 4.6.

> **Box 4.8 Summary tips for setting up a day case anaesthesia service: analgesics**
>
> **Special demands**
>
> As the patient is due to leave the hospital within hours after surgery, pain should be managed adequately prior to discharge and the pain management plan must be explained clearly explained to the patient in advance, pain medication should be prescribed and available to provide adequate pain relief at home.
>
> **Converting**
>
> The overall goal should be to secure adequate pain management with a minimum of side effects, sedation, nausea, fatigue, etc. In-hospital standard nurse or patient-provided intravenous opioid-based analgesia is not an option. Pain must be adequately handled by the patient himself/herself preferentially by oral analgesics. In procedures with known severe postoperative pain catheter techniques for provision of local anaesthesia para neural or in the wound should be considered.
>
> **Setting up**
>
> A multi-modal base pain management programme must be implemented and adequate oral rescue medication should be available.
>
> In procedures with expected more sever postoperative pain a system for continuous local anaesthesia administration via wound or para-neuronal catheter should be implemented.
>
> **Think about**
>
> As a general rule; try to block the pain signalling pathways as early as possible, all from the surgical site with local anaesthesia, peripheral acting analgesics and central-acting opioids as the top of the pyramid.

46

Further reading

Abrahams MS, Aziz MF, Fu RF Horn J-L. Ultrasound guidance compared with electrical neurostimulation for peripheral nerve block: a systematic review and meta-analysis of randomized controlled trials. *Br J Anaesthesia* 2009 **102**(3):408–17.

Apfelbaum JL, Desjardins PJ, Brown MT, Verburg KM. Multiple-day efficacy of parecoxib sodium treatment in postoperative bunionectomy pain. *Clin J Pain* 2008 Nov-Dec; **24**(9):784–92.

Capdevila X, Dadure C, Bringuier S, Bernard N, Biboulet P, Gaertner E, Macaire P. Effect of patient-controlled perineural analgesia on rehabilitation and pain after ambulatory orthopedic surgery: a multicenter randomized trial. *Anesthesiology* 2006 Sep; **105**(3): 566–73.

Capdevila X, Ponrouch M, Choquet O. Continuous peripheral nerve blocks in clinical practice. *Curr Opin Anaesthesiol.* 2008 Oct; **21**(5): 619–23. Review.

http://www.asra.com/newsletters/2000november/research_column.iphtml

Ilfeld BM, Enneking FK. Continuous peripheral nerve blocks at home: a review. *Anesth Analg* 2005 Jun; **100**(6):1822–33. Review.

Post-operative pain. Edited by David J Rowbotham Oxford Anaesthesia Library.

Sun T, Sacan O, White PF, Coleman J, Rohrich RJ, Kenkel JM. Perioperative versus postoperative celecoxib on patient outcomes after major plastic surgery procedures. *Anesth Analg* 2008 Mar; **106**(3):950–8, table of contents.

Turan I, Hein A, Jacobson E, Jakobsson JG. Sevoflurane requirement during elective ankle day surgery: the effects of etirocoxib premedication, a prospective randomised study. *J Orthop Surg Res* 2008 Sep **11**(3): 40.

White PF, Sacan O, Tufanogullari B, Eng M, Nuangchamnong N, Ogunnaike B. Effect of short-term postoperative celecoxib administration on patient outcome after outpatient laparoscopic surgery. *Can J Anaesth* 2007 May; **54**(5):342–8.

Recommended publications on regional nerve blockade

Horlocker T. Peripheral nerve blocks—regional anesthesia for the new millennium, *Regional Anesthesia and Pain Medicine.* **23**(3): 237–40.

Peripheral Nerve Blocks: A Color Atlas, third edition edited by Jacques E Chelly, published by Lippincott, Williams, & Wilkins, 2008, 496 pp.

Peripheral Nerve Blocks on DVD: Lower Limbs (from the Regional Anesthesia and Pain Medicine series) by Francis V. Salinas, published by Churchill Livingstone, 2004.

Ultrasound Guidance for Nerve Blocks: Principles and Practical Implementation by Peter Marhofer, published by Oxford University Press, 2008, 160 pp.

Atlas of Ultrasound- and Nerve Stimulation-Guided Regional Anesthesia by Ban Tsui, published by Springer Verlag, 2008, 304 pp.

Chapter 5

Anaesthetics in day case surgery

Key points

- The day surgical patient should become eligible for discharge within hours after the end of anaesthesia.
- Intravenous induction with propofol followed by maintenance with either of the third- generation inhaled anaesthetics, sevoflurane or desflurane, or propofol infusion is equally effective.
- How an anaesthetic is used is of far greater importance than which specific anaesthetic is chosen. The co-administration of an opioid should be done on an individual basis and with the lowest effective dose and should be avoided if possible.
- Avoiding higher doses of opioid and muscle relaxation maintaining spontaneous respiration enables better titration of anaesthetic, facilitates rapid recovery, and decreases the risk for PONV.
- The depth of anaesthesia monitoring may facilitate dosing and reduce the amount of the main anaesthetic and emergence in patients receiving muscle relaxants
- Selective spinal anaesthesia with low-dose bupivacaine and fentanyl has become an interesting alternative for surgery on the lower limb.
- Regional anaesthetic techniques may be an option in centres with skill in performing blocks and especially where chloroprocaine is available. Regional techniques combining intraoperative anaesthesia and postoperative analgesia by the use of catheter techniques have shown most reassuring results for more extensive surgery.

49

Day surgery covers, in general, elective "uncomplicated high volume" surgery and planning is of utmost importance, and waiting time and unnecessary delays should be minimized. Patients should be informed and prepared in advance, and time spent in holding areas should be kept as short as possible. The typical patient does not experience pain before surgery and thus the need for preoperative analgesics and anxiolytics should be limited.

5.1 **Premedication**

Adequate and professional information for and handling of the patient during preparation for surgery is of huge importance. Efforts made in order to be on time are also of great importance and reduce anxiety. Premedication can in many instances be avoided. Small doses of a benzodiazepine may be given on an individual basis. Midazolam liquid (buccal administration) is a simple and safe option if needed.

Preoperative loading with paracetamol and an NSAID/Coxib is frequently performed (see also the chapter on analgesia). The intra-operative effects of Paracetamol have not been well studied; however NSAIDs may have small but still intraoperative effects. Administering oral analgesic prior to surgery aims at facilitating awakening with a minimum of pain.

Good preoperative information and preparation can help to avoid any unnecessary delays. Realistic time planning and maintaining schedules should be aimed at.

5.2 **Induction**

Intravenous induction is simple, safe and effective. Propofol is currently the most popular induction agent. The sleep dose of propofol is decreased with a co-induction opioid. The single drug or co-induction, with small amounts of less than 1 mg doses (5–10 mcg per kg) of alfentanil, or 0.5–1 mcg per kg of fentanyl, is a matter of personal preference. Patients should be informed about the risk for pain on injection from propofol. Pre-injection of lidocaine with a rubber tourniquet before the propofol injection is the most effective regimen in order to avoid pain on injection. If available, the propofol-MCT/LCT-Emulsion is also helpful in decreasing painful propofol induction. A strategy that is adapted to the daily clinical practice should be adopted, e.g. lidocaine preinjection and the use of propofol-MCT/LCT-Emulsion. The incidence of moderate to severe local pain induced by intravenous propofol can also be decreased by a readily applicable technique in which a low dose of propofol emulsion is administered slowly by the same intravenous route 2 min in advance. This is also useful for sedation and relaxation during washing and dressing.

5.3 **Maintenance of anaesthesia**

There has been a long and intense debate about the optimal drug and route of delivery for maintenance of anaesthesia for day surgery. All the presently available alternatives are suitable; propofol continuous infusion, sevoflurane, and desflurane all have certain benefits. Isoflurane is another option, however the lower blood gas solubility associated with the use of sevoflurane and desflurane may justify their use. Table 5.1 shows the physiochemical properties of inhaled anaesthetics.

Table 5.1 Inhaled anaesthetic kinetics

	MAC in oxygen/air(%)			MAC in 67% N₂O (%)			BP (°C)	SVP (kPa)	Oil: gas part. coeff.	Blood: gas part. coeff.	MW	Biotrans. (%)
	1yr	40yr	80yr	1yr	40yr	80yr						
Halothane	0.95	0.75	0.58	0.47	0.27	0.10	50.2	32.5	224	2.3	197.4	25
Enflurane	2.08	1.63	1.27	1.03	0.58	0.22	56.5	22.9	96	1.91	184.5	3
Isoflurane	1.49	1.17	0.91	0.74	0.42	0.17	48.5	31.9	91	1.4	184.5	0.2
Sevoflurane	2.29	1.80	1.40	1.13	0.65	0.25	58.5	21.3	53	0.59	200	2.5
Desflurane	8.3	6.6	5.1	4.2	2.4	0.93	23.5	88.5	18.7	0.42	168	Minimal
Nitrous Oxide	133	104	81	NA	NA	NA	−88	5080	1.4	0.47	44	0
Xenon	92	72	57	NA	NA	NA	−107.1	5800	20	0.14	131.3	0

Potency (MAC) correlates with oil: gas partition coefficient (hence lipid solubility).
Speed of onset correlates with blood: gas partition coefficient (lower = faster).
SVP = saturated vapour pressure at 20°C, part. coeff. = partition coefficient at 37°C, MW = molecular weight, BP = boiling point, biotrans. = biotransformation

Table 5.1 is reproduced from *Oxford Handbook of Anaesthesia*, Second Edition edited by Keith G. Allman and Iain H. Wilson, (2006), with permission from Oxford University Press.

CHAPTER 5 **Anaesthetics in day case surgery**

The profound interaction between opioids and the main anaesthetic agent used should be considered in the day surgery setting also. For example, small doses of fentanyl profoundly reduce the need for the main anaesthetic agent. A minor dose of 2 mcg/kg fentanyl markedly decreases the $MAC_{tracheal\ intubation}$ for sevoflurane from 3.55 to 1.45 % Et.

In day case anaesthesia when intubation is not required and much of the surgical pain/noxious influx can be blocked by local anaesthesia, the dose of opioid should be reduced to a minimum. Co-administration of small doses of short-acting opioids reduces the need for inhaled anaesthetics without a major impact on emergence, but it may increase the risk for postoperative emesis, PONV. The opioid dose should be kept as low as possible and whenever feasible opioids should be completely avoided. In minor day case anaesthesia with sevoflurane, there may not be a need for any opioid supplementation.

The inhaled anaesthetics sevoflurane and desflurane are easy to use, their end-tidal concentrations can be monitored on-line in real-time, they have low inter-individual variations in response to noxious stimulation (ED95 is in the magnitude of 1.3 time ED50), and they are rapidly eliminated, providing quick emergence.

5.4 **Brain monitors**

Titration of the main anaesthetic agent to each individual patient's unique need, balanced against the surgical stimulation in real time, is of huge importance in day case anaesthesia. The currently available brain monitors such as BIS (Aspect Medical Systems, Inc. Norwood, USA), AAI (AEP Monitor/2™, Danmeter A/S Odense, Denmark), or CSI (Cerebral State Monitor™, Danmeter A/S Odense, Denmark) are tools that can be used to improve drug delivery and dosing, especially in patients requiring muscle relaxation and/or those taking cardiovascular drugs. All effort helping to optimize administration of main anaesthetic facilitates recovery and may have an impact on PONV.

The use of BIS or similar monitoring may reduce anaesthetic consumption. BIS-titrated anaesthesia has been shown to have an impact on the risk for PONV. The effects of duration of anaesthesia and BIS monitoring on the risk for PONV were shown once again in the ENIGMA trial results. Figure 5.1 illustrates the impact of various factors on PONV, including BIS monitoring.

The effects of brain monitoring in minor day case anaesthesia of short duration and with spontaneous breathing patients may, however, be disputed. In minor cases with spontaneous breathing, the EEG-based technique adds both unnecessary time in getting started and the added cost of the disposable electrode without providing much support in an uncomplicated case.

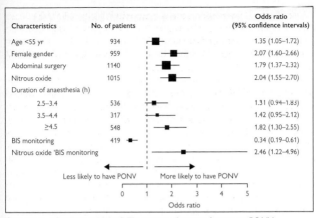

Characteristics	No. of patients		Odds ratio (95% confidence intervals)
Age <55 yr	934		1.35 (1.05–1.72)
Female gender	959		2.07 (1.60–2.66)
Abdominal surgery	1140		1.79 (1.37–2.32)
Nitrous oxide	1015		2.04 (1.55–2.70)
Duration of anaesthesia (h)			
2.5–3.4	536		1.31 (0.94–1.83)
3.5–4.4	317		1.42 (0.95–2.12)
≥4.5	548		1.82 (1.30–2.55)
BIS monitoring	419		0.34 (0.19–0.61)
Nitrous oxide 'BIS monitoring			2.46 (1.22–4.96)

Less likely to have PONV ← | → More likely to have PONV

Odds ratio: 0 1 2 3 4 5

Figure 5.1 PONV from Myles P The impact of various factors on PONV. Reproduced from Leslie K et al Risk factors for severe postoperative nausea and vomiting in a randomized trial of nitrous oxide-based vs nitrous oxide-free anaesthesia. *British Journal of Anaesthesia* **101**(4): 498–505 (2008), with permission from Oxford University Press.

The educational role of EEG-monitoring should not be forgotten. Also, in simple cases observation of the Bi-spectral index not infrequently provides new insight in the hands of the skilled anaesthetist.

The Surgical Stress Index based on heart rate and pulse oximetry amplitude has recently been described and may in future become an option. Utilizing all information that is easily available, including heart rate, respiratory rate, blood pressure, and also the pulse oximetry amplitude, to make a composite evaluation, is part of the art of day case anaesthesia.

5.5 The simple spontaneous breathing case

In the spontaneous breathing patient anaesthetized without muscle relaxants, clinical monitoring and vital signs are in most cases sufficient for the titration of optimal depth of anaesthesia. In the spontaneous breathing day case patient anaesthetized with sevoflurane or desflurane, maintaining vital signs within 20% from base line is in most patients sufficient for adequate control of depth of anaesthesia. Muscle activity, movements, increase in heart rate and/or blood pressure are obvious signs of light anaesthesia and cardiovascular depression of unnecessarily deep anaesthesia. The respiratory rate may be a valuable indicator for the potential need for additional opioid analgesia.

5.6 **Total intravenous anaesthesia (TIVA)**

Propofol was introduced over 20 years ago and has gained huge popularity. The well-established features of propofol, which provides a rapid and smooth induction and rapid and pleasant recovery after cessation of administration, makes it a first-line option for induction and also for maintenance during brief day case procedures. Propofol is associated with very minor postoperative side effects and may even exhibit antiemetic effects in low doses.

Propofol, with its fast favourable kinetics, short duration of action, and low incidence of postoperative side effects is also an attractive agent for maintenance of anaesthetic during day case surgery. The development of 'intelligent techniques' for the administration of propofol via target control kinetic pumps using a built-in algorithm for calculation of the effects-site propofol concentration, has improved continuous propofol delivery. The target control infusion (TCI) systems support optimization of intraoperative conditions and recovery, thereby allowing faster home readiness in the ambulatory setting. The definition of TCI in anaesthesia, is an infusion system which allows the anaesthetist to select the target blood concentration required for a particular effect, and then to control the depth of anaesthesia by adjusting the requested target concentration. The acronym TCI is now used as a broader term to describe the technique for the continuous control of the concentration in blood or plasma of an infused drug. TCI involves the use of a microprocessor to manage the pump. Instead of setting an infusion rate in terms of mg/kg/h, the anaesthetist enters the following:

- Body weight of the patient
- Age of the patient
- Required blood concentration of the drug (= target blood concentration in g/ml).

Today this technique is not only available for propofol but also for the administration of remifentanil, allowing total intravenous anaesthesia to be supplied by 2 TCI systems; one for control of hypnosis—propofol, and one for control of analgesia/stress—remifentanil. The TCI effect-site concentration in ASA 1–2 subjects for loss of consciousness and non-response to tenatic nerve stimuli has been studied. The effect-site EC(50) at loss of consciousness was 2.8 mcg ml($\pm$1) with an rather huge individual variation; EC(05) and EC(95) of 1.5 and 4.1 mcg ml($\pm$1), respectively. The predicted EC(50) for no response to a tetanic stimulus was 5.2 mcg ml($\pm$1) (EC(05) and EC(95) of 3.1 and 7.2 mcg ml($\pm$1), respectively). The interaction with opioid analgesics has also been determined. A profound synergistic interaction between remifentanil and propofol during surgery has been documented (Figure 5.2).

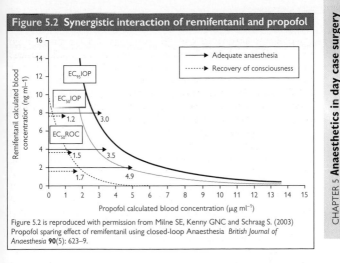

Figure 5.2 Synergistic interaction of remifentanil and propofol

Figure 5.2 is reproduced with permission from Milne SE, Kenny GNC and Schraag S. (2003) Propofol sparing effect of remifentanil using closed-loop Anaesthesia *British Journal of Anaesthesia* **90**(5): 623–9.

A dose-dependent decrease in clinical propofol requirements with increasing remifentanil concentrations has been shown. Patients were administered remifentanil to a target blood concentration of 2 ng ml±1 (low), 4 ng ml±1 (medium), or 8 ng ml±1 (high), administered by target-controlled infusion (TCI). The mean (95% CI) propofol target blood concentration during adequate anaesthesia was 4.96 (3.85–6.01) mcg ml(±1) in the low, 3.46 (2.96–3.96) mcg ml(±1) in the medium, and 3.01 (2.20–3.38) mcg ml(±1) in the high group. No significant difference was seen in recovery end points between the groups.

Propofol-based anaesthesia does not require a sophisticated anaesthetic machine and gas scavenging equipment, but merely a syringe pump and simple breathing equipment for oxygen and air mixture. Propofol-based anaesthesia has therefore become popular for sedation/anaesthesia in offices, endoscopy suits, and catheterization labs. Propofol-based anaesthesia is associated with rapid recovery and very low risk for postoperative nausea and vomiting.

The profound interaction between opioid and inhaled anaesthetics is applicable for propofol as well as for the inhaled anaesthetics sevoflurane and desflurane. This does not necessarily make it a good thing. Using more propofol/sevoflurane/desflurane is not necessarily a bad thing, but the use of opioids, especially in combination with vapours, increases the risk for PONV. The opioid dose should therefore be kept as low as possible also in combination with propofol.

5.7 Fresh gas flow and composition

The fresh gas flow must be set in order to ascertain adequate oxygenation and avoid re-breathing and CO_2 accumulation. The availability of a breathing circle that includes a CO_2 absorber will determine whether lower flows can be used or not.

Circle systems with a CO_2 absorber is strongly recommended whenever inhaled anaesthetics are to be used. Lowering the fresh-gas flow has a major impact on the amount of vapour used, subsequently reducing costs and the adverse ecological effects of waste gas release into the atmosphere. Fresh-gas flows in the magnitude of 1 L./min or less are also highly feasible for short outpatient anaesthesia in a circle system with the patients appropriately monitored with vital signs and gas monitoring; FiO_2, $EtCO_2$, and inspired as well as expired anaesthetic gas concentration. When lower flows are used vaporizer settings must be made accordingly. The dial number will be far higher than inspired (Fiaa) and close monitoring or dial, Fiaa and Etaa is recommended. The impact of the fresh gas flow, volume and composition is illustrated in Figure 5.3.

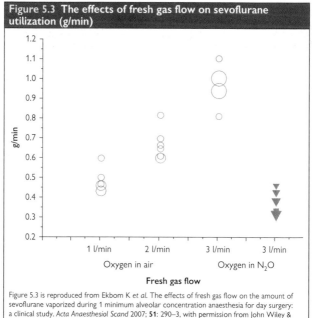

Figure 5.3 The effects of fresh gas flow on sevoflurane utilization (g/min)

Figure 5.3 is reproduced from Ekbom K *et al.* The effects of fresh gas flow on the amount of sevoflurane vaporized during 1 minimum alveolar concentration anaesthesia for day surgery: a clinical study. *Acta Anaesthesiol Scand* 2007; **51**: 290–3, with permission from John Wiley & Sons, Inc.

The composition of fresh gas has been the subject of extensive discussion. The use of nitrous oxide as part of the fresh gas flow reduces the need for main anaesthetic, facilitates spontaneous respiration, and shortens emergence. The use of nitrous oxide remains an option and reduces the need for a "second, main anaesthetic". For all the commonly used main anaesthetics, sevoflurane, desflurane and propofol, consumption is significantly reduced when nitrous oxide is used. The influence of nitrous oxide on PONV is rather limited. In a large analysis of various factors on PONV by Apfel et al., no significant difference was shown between fresh gas consisting of oxygen and air compared with oxygen and nitrous oxide (see Figure 5.4).

The potential benefits of high-inspired concentrations of oxygen on PONV have been described but the evidence for its effect is lacking. The positive impact of a high-inspired oxygen fraction on surgical site wound infection may not be relevant for day surgery.

5.8 Which agent?

Many studies have looked at the effects of the main anaesthetic. The characteristics of the ideal agent are listed in Table 5.2.

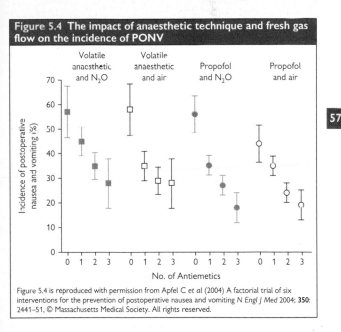

Figure 5.4 The impact of anaesthetic technique and fresh gas flow on the incidence of PONV

Figure 5.4 is reproduced with permission from Apfel C et al (2004) A factorial trial of six interventions for the prevention of postoperative nausea and vomiting N Engl J Med 2004; **350**: 2441–51, © Massachusetts Medical Society. All rights reserved.

The pharmacological features of the inhaled anaesthetics and the evolution of their clinical introduction are summarized in Table 5.3.

The choice of main anaesthetic in clinical practice, sevoflurane, desflurane, or propofol, seems, however, not to have major impact on the outcome.

In the morbidly obese patient, desflurane may exhibit some advantages due to its lower solubility in blood as well as in fat tissues. Many protocols for bariatric surgery include desflurane for maintenance of anaesthesia (see also *Anaesthesia for the Overweight and Obese Patient* by Mark Bellamy and Michel Struys published in the same series).

For the average day case procedure, differences may be seen in emergence (Table 5.4 and 5.5).

Table 5.2 Properties of an ideal anaesthetic for ambulatory surgery

- Pleasant, rapid and smooth onset of effect, without pain or irritating colour
- Provided hypnosis, amnesia, analgesia and muscle relaxation sufficient for surgery
- Intra-operative side effects (e.g. cardiovascular instability, respiratory depression, spontaneous movements, or excitatory activity) absent or minimal
- Rapid recovery profile without postoperative side effects (especially nausea, vomiting, dizziness and shivering)
- Easy to titrate for increased or decreased depth of anaesthesia
- Provides residual analgesia during the early postoperative period
- Cost-effective

Table 5.2 is reproduced from Ghatge S, Lee J and Smith I. Sevoflurane: an ideal agent for adult day-case anesthesia? *Acta Anaesthesiol Scand* 2003; **47**: 917–31, with permission from John Wiley & Sons, Inc.

Table 5.3 Properties of the currently available inhaled anaesthetic agents

	Halothane	Enflurane	Isoflurane	Desflurane	Sevoflurane
Introduced	1956	1971	1980	1993	1995*
Boiling point (°C)	50.2	56.5	48.5	23.5	58.5
Blood gas solubility	2.5	1.9	1.4	0.42	0.69
Vapour solubility	32.1	23.3	32.5	89.2	22.7
°C (Kpa) MAC (%)	0.75	1.7	1.15	6	2.05
Induction characteristics	Smooth, slow, dysrhythmias common	Irritable	Irritable	Very irritable; not recommended	Smooth acceptably rapid

Table 5.3 (*Contd.*)

	Halothane	Enflurane	Isoflurane	Desflurane	Sevoflurane
Cardiac stability	Depressant dysrhythmias common, sensitizes heart to epinephrine	Depressant some tachycardia	Depressant some tachycardia	Mild depressant, stimulation with concentration increases	Mild depressant, normal heart rate
Ease of titration	Limited by solubility	Limited by potency	Limited by irritability	Limited by irritability	Facilitated by insolubility and lack of irritation
Early recovery	Slow	Moderate	Moderate	Rapid	Rapid after short procedures
Metabolism (%)	20	2	0.2	0.02	5

Table 5.3 is reproduced from Ghatge S, Lee J and Smith I. Sevoflurane: an ideal agent for adult day-case anesthesia? *Acta Anaesthesiol Scand* 2003; **47**: 917–31, with permission from John Wiley & Sons, Inc.

Table 5.4 Patient demographics and perioperative observations

	Propofol (n= 34)	Desflurane (n = 34)	Sevoflurane (n = 34)
Age (yr)	46 ± 13	43 ± 12	47 ± 11
Weight (kg)	77 ± 14	78 ± 13	80 ± 14
Duration anaesthesia (min)	17 ± 6 (7–35)	18 ± 5 (10–35)	19 ± 8 (9–39)
Duration surgery (min)	14 ± 5 (6–28)	17 ± 5 (8–33)	18 ± 7 (6–38)
Time to laryngeal mask removal (min)	4.7 ± 1.9*** (1–9)	2.7 ± 0.8 (1–4)	3.2 ± 1.1 (1–6)
Time to state birthdate (min)	6.4 ± 2.6*** (2–15)	3.4 ± 1.0 (1–6)	3.9 ± 1.2 (1–6)
VAS 30 min	1.7 ± 2.7	0.8 ± 2.0	1.0 ± 1.9
VAS 60 min	2.8 ± 2.4	1.7 ± 2.4	1.6 ± 2.2
PONV (n)	1	1	3
Discharge time (min)	65 ± 23	55 ± 19	56 ± 18

Table 5.4 is reproduced from Dolk, A et al. Inhalation anaesthesia is cost-effective for ambulatory surgery: a clinical comparison with propofol during elective knee arthroscopy. *European Journal of Anaesthesiology* 2002; **19**: 88–92, with permission from Cambridge University Press.

Looking at recovery from a more protracted perspective, quality of recovery, and discharge time, the anaesthetic drug chosen seems to be of minor importance (Table 5.6)

It was concluded in a recent meta-analysis of inhaled anaesthetics that meta-analysis of studies in which the duration of aneasthesia was up to 3.1 hours indicated that patients receiving either desflurane or sevoflurane did not exhibit significant differences in PACU time or PONV frequency. Patients receiving desflurane followed commands, were extubated, and were oriented earlier than patients receiving sevoflurane (see Table 5.5).

Table 5.5 Differences between sevoflurane and desflurane in operating room recovery times

| | Difference in outcome (Sevoflurane—Desflurane) (min)[a] | |
Obeyed Commands (Mean ± S.E.)	Extubated (Mean ± S.E.)	Oriented (Mean ± S.E.)
3.8 ± 1.5	3.1 ± 1.0	1.9 ± 1.6
8.7 ± 1.1	NR	13.0 ± 1.7
1.6 ± 1.1	1.2 ± 1.4	2.7 ± 1.5
2.2 ± 0.6	1.9 ± 0.7	1.8 ± 1.0
NR	2.8 ± 1.4	NR
NR	NR	4.9 ± 1.1
0.5 ± 0.6	0.5 ± 0.7	1.5 ± 1.0
0.0 ± 0.4	NR	2.0 ± 0.6
2.0 ± 0.5	NR	2.0 ± 0.8
0.0 ± 0.5	0.0 ± 0.5	NR
0.4 ± 2.0	3.5 ± 1.9	NR
NR	9.1 ± 2.9	NR
−2.0 ± 1.2	−3.0 ± 1.3	−3.0 ± 1.4
0.0 ± 1.2	−1.0 ± 1.3	−1.0 ± 1.4
−0.6 ± 1.6	0.5 ± 0.9	0.9 ± 1.3
1.3 ± 0.8	0.8 ± 1.2	0.8 ± 1.2
4.0 ± 1.9	4.0 ± 1.3	NR
4.5 ± 1.3	1.5 ± 0.8	3.3 ± 1.4
NR	NR	0.0 ± 1.6
NR	2.8 ± 4.3	NR
NR	NR	0.5 ± 0.3
1.8±0.6	NR	1.8 ± 0.8

Table 5.5 is reproduced with permission from Macario et al. (2005) Meta-analysis of trials comparing postoperative recovery after anaesthesia with sevoflurane or desflurane. *American Journal of Health-System Pharmacy*, **62**: 63–8.

Table 5.6 Differences between sevoflurane and desflurane in PACU recovery times[a]

	Difference in Outcome (Sevoflurane—Desflurane) (min)[b]
Phase I PACU Discharge (Mean ± S.E.)	Ready for Discharge Home (Mean ± S.E.)
−10.0 ± 0.5	−8.0 ± 22.9
NR	−8.0 ± 12.9
−2.0 ± 3.1	2.0 ± 17.3
2.0 ± 3.3	−8.0 ± 20.5
−7.5 ± 9.3	NR
NR	21.0 ± 16.1
−6.0 ± 1.5	3.0 ± 9.9
−7.0 ± 1.0	−11.0 ± 14.4
3.0 ± 1.4	−38.0 ± 12.2
−10.0 ± 11.5	−15.0 ± 13.8
−8.0 ± 8.0	−23.0 ± 21.8
7.0 ± 7.9	51.0 ± 17.7
−2.0 ± 14.5	NR
28.0 ± 18.5	NR
NR	2.0 ± 15.1
NR	2 ± 53.0
NR	1 ± 4.5
NR	−3.0 ± 4.4
4.1 ± 9.3	NR

Table 5.6 is reproduced with permission from Macario et al. (2005) Meta-analysis of trials comparing postoperative recovery after anaesthesia with sevoflurane or desflurane, American Journal of Health-System Pharmacy, 62: 63 8.

Also, when total intravenous anaesthesia (TIVA) and volatile induction and maintenance of anaesthesia (VIMA) is taken into account no major differences can be seen in the outcome.

Also, when isoflurane is included as main anaesthetic and compared to sevoflurane, desflurane, and propofol for maintenance of anaesthesia Gupta et al. in their systematic review, "Comparison of recovery profile after ambulatory anaesthesia with propofol, isoflurane, sevoflurane and desflurane" concluded: "the choice of anaesthetic for maintenance of anaesthesia should be guided by the training and experience of the individual physician, as well as the routines and equipment available in the hospital, because the specific anaesthetic appears to play a minor role in outcome after ambulatory surgery."

Skill and experience in use and handling, and optimization of administration, is however of outmost importance.

Numerous studies have been conducted comparing the main anaesthetics for day case anaesthesia: propofol, sevoflurane and desflurane. All three are easy to use with spontaneous breathing and a laryngeal mask airway (see Table 5.4). It seems reasonable to conclude that all are safe and efficacious. Desflurane, with its lower solubility in blood as well as other body compartments, is in most studies associated with a more rapid emergence and regain of cognitive function (see Table 5.5). However, the time to ready for discharge is dependent on a variety of factors and the impact of the main anaesthetic is not that important (see Table 5.6). Also, when propofol and isoflurane are used no major differences are seen in more protracted recovery variables (see Tables 5.7 and 5.8).

Table 5.7 Mental state and nausea and vomiting in recovery and on the postoperative ward-by-randomization group

Outcome	Group P/P (n=265)	Group P/I (n=267)	Group P/S (n=280)	Group S/S (n=251)
Recovery:				
Postoperative nausea and vomiting (PONV) in the recovery room				
None	244 (92%)	240 (90%)	252 (90%)	201 (80%)
Nausea	19 (7%)	24 (9%)	27 (10%)	34 (14%)
One emetic episode	2 (1%)	3 (1%)	0 (0%)	12 (5%)
Multiple emetic episodes	0 (0%)	0 (0%)	1 (0.5%)	4 (1%)
Cumulative PONV in recovery	21 (8%)	27 (10%)	28 (10%)	50 (20%)*
Mental state				
Alert and awake	158 (60%)	158 (59%)	163 (58%)	140 (56%)
Agitated and distressed	15 (6%)	21 (8%)	13 (5%)	19 (7%)
Drowsy	91 (34%)	88 (33%)	101 (36%)	87 (35%)
Missing	1 (0.5%)	0 (0%)	3 (1%)	5 (2%)
Postoperative ward:				
PONV on the postoperative ward				
None	246 (93%)	232 (87%)	248 (89%)	202 (80%)
Nausea	15 (6%)	22 (8%)	19 (7%)	36 (14%)

Table 5.7 (Contd.)

Outcome	Group P/P (n=265)	Group P/I (n=267)	Group P/S (n=280)	Group S/S (n=251)
One emetic episode	3 (1%)	6 (2%)	5 (2%)	9 (4%)
Multiple emetic episodes	1 (0.5%)	7 (3%)	6 (2%)	4 (2%)
Cumulative PONV on ward	19 (7%)	35 (13%)	30 (11%)	49 (20%)
* P <0.01 compared with Group P/P (Fisher's exact test).				
Recovery time	41.1 (38.6–43.6)	40.4 (37.9–42.8)	41.1 (38.7–43.4)	42.4 (39.5–45.4)
Time to discharge	320.8 (243.3–398.3)	345.8 (264.4–427.2)	316.8 (239.7–393.85)	330.3 (242.9–368.4)

Table 5.7 is reproduced with permission from Moore et al. (2008) The effect of anaesthesia agents on induction, recovery and patient preferences in adult day case surgery: a 7-day follow-up randomized controlled trial. *European Journal of Anaesthesiology*, **25**: 876–83.

Table 5.8 Post-discharge recovery-by-randomization group

Outcome		Group P/P (n=265)	Group P/I (n=267)	Group P/S (n=280)	Group S/S (n=251)
Presence of postoperative pain*	Day 1$^\alpha$	94 (35%)	95 (36%)	96 (34%)	93 (37%)
	Day 7$^\beta$	41 (15%)	43 (16%)	39 (14%)	42 (17%)
Difficulty concentrating*	Day 1$^\gamma$	51 (19%)	47 (18%)	48 (17%)	54 (22%)
	Day 7$^\delta$	10 (4%)	11 (4%)	13 (5%)	13 (5%)
Forgetfulness*	Day 1	41 (15%)	34 (13%)	34 (17%)	41 (17%)
	Day 7$^\xi$	15 (6%)	12 (4%)	34 (17%)	43 (17%)
Return (actual and estimated) to normal activities—mean days (n)$^\$$		6.8 (n = 183)	64 (n =179)	6.6 (n = 171)	6.3 (n = 160)

Table 5.8 is reproduced with permission from Moore et al. (2008) The effect of anaesthesia agents on induction, recovery and patient preferences in adult day case surgery: a 7-day follow-up randomized controlled trial. *European Journal of Anaesthesiology*, **25**: 876–83.

5.9 **Regional anaesthesia in day case surgery**

Spinal anaesthesia has had a long history of use for surgery of the lower part of the body. Lidocaine spinal anaesthesia was a most suitable technique providing rapid onset of block and rapid recovery of motor function. Because of the concerns for transient neurologic symptoms after the use of lidocaine 50 mg/ml, many countries have since withdrawn lidocaine for spinal use. Alternatives have been sought. Low-dose bupivacaine with or without fentanyl supplementation has been shown to be effective for knee arthroscopy, providing effective intraoperative anaesthesia and rapid recovery. Eligiblity for discharge using bupivacaine has been shown to be reached similar to desflurane general anaesthesia.

The selective "unilateral" spinal blocks have also been shown to reduce the decrease in blood pressure commonly seen following traditional spinal blocks. The unilateral, selective spinal with rapid onset and offset of action with a minimum of hemodynamic alterations makes it an interesting option in more fragile patients, for example those with cardiovascular disease.

In countries where available chloroprocaine seems to be an interesting alternative, doses of 35–50 mg of chloroprocaine 10 mg/ml have been shown to provide satisfactory anaesthesia with rapid offset of both sensory and motor block. Patients receiving chloroprocaine were eligible for discharge with 2 hours.

Low-dose, "selective spinal anaesthesia" has become an interesting alternative to general anaesthesia in the day case setting also, especially for surgery of the lower limb (i.e., knee, ankle and foot surgery). It is also an interesting alternative for surgery in the prone position, especially in cases where the body position needs to be changed repeatedly (e.g., extensive varicose veins). Low dose spinal anaesthesia has also been shown to be feasible for use in lower abdominal laparoscopic surgery.

5.10 **Plexus and other peripheral blocks**

Plexus and other peripheral blocks are techniques not only in order to provide postoperative pain relief, but also for intraoperative anaesthesia and especially for surgery on the extremities (arm/hand lower limb/ankle/foot). The use of plexus and peripheral blocks should, of course, take into account the skill required for satisfactory performance of the block, time to onset, and the potential for failed/partial-failed block.

Ultrasound guided techniques improve success rates to a major extent, but implementation of the technique carries with it investment in time and equipment. All the standard local anaesthetics can be used.

The use of chloroprocaine enables a somewhat more rapid onset and offset of the block, facilitating the use in day case anaesthesia.

(See also Chapter 4 Analgesics on day surgery and the section on Regional analgesia.)

5.11 **Intravenous regional anaesthesia (IVRA): the Bier block**

Intravenous regional anaesthesia (IVRA) is an option for day case procedures on the arm below the elbow or leg below the knee that will be completed within 40–60 minutes. This simple method of providing anaesthesia of the distal arm or leg was first described by August Bier in 1808. IVRA is safe and efficacious when used in accordance with accepted national standards. Onset of anaesthesia is acceptably rapid; 20–25 minutes should be allowed in order to obtain

---

Box 5.1 Summary tips for setting up a day case anaesthesia service: anaesthetics in day surgery

Special demands

Day surgical patients must be ascertained to have safe and efficacious anaesthesia, but should recover and be able to leave hospital safely within hours after the end of anaesthesia. Anaesthetic techniques, drug or drug combinations providing smooth onset, safe intraoperative course, and minimal residual anaesthetic effects, should be sought.

Converting

Liberal use of opioids and or muscle relaxants must be avoided. Balanced anaesthesia, combining drugs facilitating rapid recovery is warranted.

Setting up

Anaesthetic administration, fine-tuning of administration to achieve excellence and tailoring the administration of anaesthesia to each patient's unique need in real time is of more importance than drug choice. It is more how you use, administer, and titrate drugs, than which specific drugs are used that will provide success.

Think about

Day case anaesthesia is a process of fine-tuning, watching the surgeon, and being one step ahead. Plan for incision. Plan for emergence in conjunction with wound closure. Successful day case anaesthesia/surgery is a team effort.

a good nerve block and so that reasonable muscle relaxation can be obtained. The use of IVRA should be limited to procedures lasting less than 1 hour because of increasing discomfort from the tourniquet. The drug of choice for IVRA is prilocaine, as it is the least toxic local anaesthetic and as it has the largest therapeutic index. If prilocaine is not available, lidocaine is an acceptable alternative. The addition of adjuncts such as clonidine or ketamine have been tested. The addition of clonidine 1 mcg/kg or ketamine 0.1 mg/kg to lidocaine for IVRA delays the onset of unbearable tourniquet pain and decreases analgesic consumption for tourniquet pain relief.

Further reading

Anaesthesia for the Elderly (Oxford Anaesthesia Library series). by Chris Dodds, Chandra M. Kumar and Frederique Servin. Oxford University Press, 2007.

Anaesthesia for the Overweight and Obese Patient (Oxford Anaesthesia Library series). Mark Bellamy and Michel Struys. Oxford University Press, 2007.

Assareh H, Anderson RE, Uusijärvi J, Jakobsson J. Sevoflurane requirements during ambulatory surgery: a clinical study with and without AEP-index guidance. *Acta Anaesthesiol Scand.* 2002 May; **46**(5): 495–9.

Bergland A, Gislason H, Raeder J. Fast-track surgery for bariatric laparoscopic gastric bypass with focus on anaesthesia and peri-operative care. Experience with 500 cases. *Acta Anaesthesiol Scand.* 2008 Nov; **52**(10): 1394–9.

Casati A, Fanelli G, Aldegheri G, Colnaghi E, Casaletti E, Cedrati V, Torri G. Frequency of hypotension during conventional or asymmetric hyperbaric spinal block. *Reg Anesth Pain Med.* 1999 May–Jun; **24**(3): 214–9.

Casati A, Fanelli G, Beccaria P, Aldegheri G, Berti M, Senatore R, Torri G. Block distribution and cardiovascular effects of unilateral spinal anaesthesia by 0.5% hyperbaric bupivacaine. A clinical comparison with bilateral spinal block. *Minerva Anestesiol.* 1998 Jul-Aug; **64**(7–8): 307–12.

Casati A, Fanelli G, Danelli G, Berti M, Ghisi D, Brivio M, Putzu M, Barbagallo A. Spinal anesthesia with lidocaine or preservative-free 2-chloroprocaine for outpatient knee arthroscopy: a prospective, randomized, double-blind comparison. *Anesth Analg.* 2007 Apr; **104**(4): 959–64.

Cuvas O, Gulec H, Karaaslan M, Basar H. The use of low dose plain solutions of local anaesthetic agents for spinal anaesthesia in the prone position: bupivacaine compared with levobupivacaine. *Anaesthesia.* 2009 Jan; **64**(1): 14–8.

Daruwalla ZJ, Halpenny M, Mullett H. Day case shoulder surgery: satisfactory pain control without regional anaesthesia. A prospective analysis of a perioperative protocol. *Ir J Med Sci.* 2008 Nov 13. [Epub ahead of print].

Dolk A, Cannerfelt R, Anderson RE, Jakobsson J.Inhalation anaesthesia is cost-effective for ambulatory surgery: a clinical comparison with propofol during elective knee arthroscopy. *Eur J Anaesthesiol.* 2002 Feb; **19**(2): 88–92.

Gupta A, Stierer T, Zuckerman R, Sakima N, Parker SD, Fleisher LA. Comparison of recovery profile after ambulatory anesthesia with propofol, isoflurane, sevoflurane and desflurane: a systematic review. *Anesth Analg.* 2004 Mar; **98**(3): 632–41.

Hadzic A, Arliss J, Kerimoglu B, Karaca PE, Yufa M, Claudio RE, Vloka JD, Rosenquist R, Santos AC, Thys DM. A comparison of infraclavicular nerve block versus general anesthesia for hand and wrist day-case surgeries. *Anesthesiology.* 2004 Jul; **101**(1): 127–32.

Hendrickx JF, Eger EI 2nd, Sonner JM, Shafer SL. Is synergy the rule? A review of anesthetic interactions producing hypnosis and immobility. *Anesth Analg.* 2008 Aug; **107**(2): 494–506. Review.

Katoh T, Nakajima Y, Moriwaki G, Kobayashi S, Suzuki A, Iwamoto T, Bito H, Ikeda K. Sevoflurane requirements for tracheal intubation with and without fentanyl. *Br J Anaesth.* 1999 Apr; **82**(4): 561–5.

Korhonen AM, Valanne JV, Jokela RM, Ravaska P, Korttila KT. A comparison of selective spinal anesthesia with hyperbaric bupivacaine and general anesthesia with desflurane for outpatient knee arthroscopy. *Anesth Analg* 2004 Dec; **99**(6): 1668–73.

Korhonen AM, Valanne JV, Jokela RM, Ravaska P, Korttila K. Intrathecal hyperbaric bupivacaine 3 mg + fentanyl 10 microg for outpatient knee arthroscopy with tourniquet. *Acta Anaesthesiol Scand.* 2003 Mar; **47**(3): 342–6.

Lennox PH, Vaghadia H, Henderson C, Martin L, Mitchell GW. Small-dose selective spinal anesthesia for short-duration outpatient laparoscopy: recovery characteristics compared with desflurane anesthesia. *Anesth Analg.* 2002 Feb; **94**(2): 346–50.

Leslie K, Myles PS, Chan MT, Paech MJ, Peyton P, Forbes A, McKenzie D; ENIGMA Trial Group. Risk factors for severe postoperative nausea and vomiting in a randomized trial of nitrous oxide-based vs nitrous oxide-free anaesthesia. *Br J Anaesth.* 2008 Oct; **101**(4): 498–505.

Liu SS. Effects of Bispectral Index monitoring on ambulatory anesthesia: a meta-analysis of randomized controlled trials and a cost analysis. *Anesthesiology.* 2004 Aug; **101**(2): 311–5.

Moore JK, Elliott RA, Payne K, Moore EW, St Leger AS, Harper NJ, Pollard BJ, Kerr J. The effect of anaesthetic agents on induction, recovery and patient preferences in adult day case surgery: a 7-day follow-up randomized controlled trial. *Eur J Anaesthesiol.* 2008 Nov; **25**(11): 876–83.

Nelskylä KA, Yli-Hankala AM, Puro PH, Korttila KT. Sevoflurane titration using bispectral index decreases postoperative vomiting in phase II recovery after ambulatory surgery. *Anesth Analg.* 2001 Nov; **93**(5): 1165–9.

Saros GB, Doolke A, Anderson RE, Jakobsson JG. Desflurane vs. sevoflurane as the main inhaled anaesthetic for spontaneous breathing via a laryngeal mask for varicose vein day surgery: a prospective randomized study. *Acta Anaesthesiol Scand.* 2006 May; **50**(5): 549–52.

Sell A, Tein T, Pitkänen M. Spinal 2-chloroprocaine: effective dose for ambulatory surgery. *Acta Anaesthesiol Scand.* 2008 May; **52**(5): 695–9.

Smith I, Walley G, Bridgman S. Omitting fentanyl reduces nausea and vomiting, without increasing pain, after sevoflurane for day surgery. *Eur J Anaesthesiol.* 2008 Oct; **25**(10): 790–9.

Wennervirta J, Hynynen M, Koivusalo AM, Uutela K, Huiku M, Vakkuri A. Surgical stress index as a measure of nociception/antinociception balance during general anesthesia. *Acta Anaesthesiol Scand.* 2008 Sep; **52**(8): 1038–45.

Chapter 6

Muscle relaxation in day case surgery

Key points

- Day case procedures in general consist of elective non-major surgerical procedures; thus, most patients are eligible for spontaneous breathing during general anaesthesia.
- Intubate and use relaxants only when there is a good reason to and avoid muscle relaxants wherever possible.
- Neuromuscular relaxation should be used only when considered necessary in day case anaesthesia.
- The role of suxamethonium may be obvious for rapid sequence induction in the emergent situation, but its place in elective day case anaesthesia is rather limited.
- When necessary use an non-depolarizing agent appropriate to the likely duration of need for relaxation and ensure good reversal.
- Neuromuscular monitoring reversed before the patient awakens is strongly recommended in order to minimize the risk for residual block.
- The availability of sugammadex opens up the possibility to maintain deep neuromuscular (rocuronium) block and still have a rapid and effective reversal within a short time.

Day case surgical procedures generally consist of elective non-major surgical procedures; therefore, most patients are eligible for spontaneous breathing during general anaesthesia.

Muscle relaxation should be avoided whenever possible. Muscle relaxation may of course be required in abdominal cases and in order to facilitate intubation when necessary. Intubation may, however, also be achieved with propofol, remifentanil, or by deepening the sevoflurane anaesthesia only. When the patient is intubated, there may not be an absolute need for muscle relaxation, as many patients are able to ventilate spontaneously adequately also on tube.

The ideal neuromuscular blocking agents for ambulatory anaesthesia are not yet available. Suxamethonium exerts a beneficial profile with regards to onset and offset of action but after-suxamethonium myalgia is seen frequently. For the competitive, non-depolarizing agents offset is slower and residual curarization following the use of curare-like agents may complicate recovery.

The only depolarizing neuromuscular blocking agent, suxamethonium, is still widely used because of its rapid onset and short duration of action, producing excellent intubating conditions, despite its numerous adverse effects. The risk for malignant hyperthermia and suxamethonium myalgia should be acknowledged. Higher suxamethonium dosage has been suggested to be followed by lower incidence of myalgia. The relationship between fasciculation and myalgia is unclear. Sodium channel blockers or non-steroidal anti-inflammatory drugs may prevent occurrence of myalgia.

Muscle relaxants with steroid structure (pancuronium, vecuronium, rocuronium) are all mainly eliminated by liver metabolism followed by biliary and partially urine excretion. The currently available benzylisoquinoliniums, including atracurium, mivacurium, and cisatracurium, are all undergoing plasma hydrolysis. The clinical profile of such agents is shown in Table 6.1.

Table 6.1 Features of non-depolarizing agents

	Onset/ duration of action	Ganglion blockade	Histamine release	Cardiac effects	Elimination
Tubo-curarine	Slow/long	Yes +++	Yes +++	Hypotension	Renal
Gallamine	Slow/long	No	No	Tachycardia	Renal
Pancuronium	Slow/long	No	No	Tachycardia	Renal/ hepatic
Vecuronium	Slow/ Intermediate	No	No	Nil	Hepatic/ renal
Atracurium	Slow/ Intermediate	No	Yes +	No	Hofmann
Mivacurium	Slow/short	No	Yes +	No	Plasma cholinesterase
Rocuronium	Rapid/ intermediate	No	No	No	Hepatic/ renal

Table 6.1 is reproduced from Thandia R. Neuromuscular blocking drugs: discovery and development . *J R Soc Med* 2002; **95**: 363–7, © Royal Society of Medicine.

There is no obvious drug of choice for muscle relaxation in day case anaesthesia. Both mivacurium and rocuronium are alternatives for short procedures.

Women are slightly more sensitive than men to rocuronium. This suggests that the routine dose of rocuronium should be somewhat reduced in women. It has also been suggested that the duration of action of rocuronium is influenced by the time of day of administration; this effect is, however, of seemingly limited clinical significance and has more practical relevance to research.

Rapacuronium initially seemed to offer some benefits compared with the currently available neuromuscular blocking agents for day care anaesthesia; however, due to the occurrence of anaphylaxis and histamine release, it has been withdrawn in most countries.

A survey of praxis in day case anaesthesia shows a rather conservative profile.

Suxamethonium was used for intubation in 8.8% patients; the three most common nondepolarizing neuromuscular blocking agents were atracurium, cisatracurium, and vecuronium.

6.1 Residual muscle weakness after curarization

Non-depolarizing neuromuscular agents have been shown to be associated with an increased risk of postoperative residual block. To reduce the risk of residual block, neuromuscular monitoring is highly advisable. The use of neostigmine for reversal and the measurement of the train of four (TOF) ratio during recovery are strongly recommended after administration of intermediate-acting neuromuscular blocking agents.

6.2 Reversal agents

The administration of reversal neostigmine and atropine has been suggested to potentially increase the risk for PONV. In a recent meta-analysis, the combination of neostigmine with either atropine or glycopyrrolate was not found to significantly increase the incidence of overall (0–24 h) vomiting (relative risk, 0.91; 95% confidence interval, 0.70–1.18; P = 0.48) or nausea. The use of reversal agents should not be restricted. Omitting reversal introduces a potential risk of residual paralysis (i.e., impaired laryngeal and pharyngeal muscle function, alterations in hypoxic ventilatory control), thus subsequently giving rise to a reduced margin of safety. A TOF ratio of > or = 0.9 is now accepted as the index of adequate recovery of neuromuscular function, and neuromuscular recovery should be routinely monitored in ambulatory patients and residual paralysis prevented by reversing neuromuscular block.

6.3 **New alternatives: sugammadex**

Sugammadex was approved by the EMEA in July 2008. It selectively reverses the neuromuscular blockade induced by rocuronium. Sugammadex does not involve inhibition of acetylcholinesterase and the autonomic instability produced by anticholinesterases, such as neostigmine and antimuscarinic agents, such as atropine, is not seen. Its administration is therefore associated with less cardiovascular and autonomic instability than the traditional reversal agents.

Studies on sugammadex have been shown to provide dose dependent effects. Sugammadex will therefore allow deep levels of block to be maintained until the very end of surgery, and will allow block to be reversed at any time after rocuronium administration, even just a few minutes. Doses of 2–16 mg/kg-1 are recommended depending on the level of block.

In one recent study increasing doses of sugammadex dose-dependently reduce the mean recovery time from 122 min (spontaneous recovery) to less than 2 min. Signs of recurrence of blockade were not observed. No serious adverse events related to sugammadex were reported. Recovery from profound rocuronium-induced neuromuscular blockade has also been shown to be significantly faster with sugammadex as opposed to neostigmine. Most of the patients receiving sugammadex (97%) recovered to a TOF ratio of 0.9 within 5 min after administration. In contrast, most patients receiving neostigmine (73%) recovered between 30 and 60 min after administration, with 23% requiring more than 60 min to recover to a TOF ratio of 0.9.

The exact role of sugammadex in routine day case anaesthesia needs to be further evaluated. The availability of sugammadex reversal may, however, increase the use of rocuronium, and decrease the need for suxamethonium.

> **Box 6.1 Summary tips for setting up a day case anaesthesia service: muscle relaxation**
>
> **Special demands**
>
> None, the day case patient only requires muscle relaxation infrequently, and muscle relaxation should be avoided as far as possible.
>
> **Converting**
>
> Critically evaluate if muscle relaxation is needed.
>
> **Setting up**
>
> Talk to the surgeon and discuss whether muscle relaxation is of critical need or not.
>
> **Think about**
>
> Muscle relaxation has a number of effects with a major impact on day case anaesthesia; patient can't breathe—needs to be ventilated, can't move/shows signs of inadequate anaesthesia, needs to be more closely observed, residual partial paralysis may negatively influence recovery.

Further reading

Adamus M, Koutna J, Gabrhelik T, Hubackova M, Janaskova E. Influence of gender on the onset and duration of rocuronium-induced neuromuscular block. *Biomed Pap Med Fac Univ Palacky Olomouc Czech Repub* 2007 Dec; **151**(2): 301–5.

Bettelli G.Which muscle relaxants should be used in day surgery and when? *Curr Opin Anaesthesiol* 2006 Dec; **19**(6): 600–5. Review.

Bowman WC. Neuromuscular block. *Br J Pharmacol* 2006; **147**: S277–S286.

Caldwell JE, Miller RD. Clinical implications of sugammadex. *Anaesthesia*. 2009 Mar; **64** Suppl 1: 66–72.

Cheesman JF, Merry AF, Pawley MD, de Souza RL, Warman GR. The effect of time of day on the duration of neuromuscular blockade elicited by rocuronium. *Anaesthesia* 2007 Nov; **62**(11): 1114–20.

Cheng CR, Sessler DI, Apfel CC. Does neostigmine administration produce a clinically important increase in postoperative nausea and vomiting? *Anesth Analg*. 2005 Nov; **101**(5): 1349–55.

de Boer HD, Driessen JJ, Marcus MA, Kerkkamp H, Heeringa M, Fuchs-Buder T, Mencke T. Use of reversal agents in day care procedures (with special reference to postoperative nausea and vomiting). *Eur J Anaesthesiol Suppl*. 2001; **23**: 53–9.

Jones RK, Caldwell JE, Brull SJ, Soto RG. Reversal of profound rocuronium-induced blockade with sugammadex: a randomized comparison with neostigmine. *Anesthesiology*. 2008 Nov; **109**(5): 816–24.

Klimek M. Reversal of rocuronium-induced (1.2 mg/kg) profound neuro-muscular block by sugammadex: a multicenter, dose-finding and safety study. *Anesthesiology* 2007 Aug; **107**(2): 239–44.

Thandia R. Neuromuscular blocking drugs: discovery and development. *J R Soc Med* 2002; **95**: 363–7.

Tramèr MR, Fuchs-Buder T. Omitting antagonism of neuromuscular block: effect on postoperative nausea and vomiting and risk of residual paralysis. A systematic review. *Br J Anaesth* 1999 Mar; **82**(3): 379–86.

Chapter 7

Airway and ventilation in day case anaesthesia

Key points

- Day surgery, in general, covers elective non-major surgery, thus spontaneous breathing and minimally invasive/traumatic airways should be considered.

- The laryngeal mask airway (LMA) or disposable alternatives should be considered in most cases of elective day surgical anaesthesia where no obvious contraindications are seen. The LMA is a safe and feasible alternative both to an ordinary facemask and to intubation in cases when the risk for regurgitation and aspiration is minor. Supra-glottic airways, such as ProSeal LMA, appear to provide effective ventilation during laparoscopy also, although their ability to protect against aspiration is still unclear.

- Spontaneous breathing is the preferred ventilation in uncomplicated day surgical anaesthesia; respiratory depression from large doses of opioids and the use of muscle relaxants should be avoided.

- Controlled mechanical ventilation should be used when deemed necessary; ventilator settings should be done in accordance to normal in-hospital practice.

- Intubation should always be readily available as a plan for failed intubation.

Securing an adequate airway and ventilation is of utmost importance in day case anaesthesia/sedation as elsewhere in anaesthesia.

The safe and efficacious management of the airway is one of most important parts of anaesthesia in general. Securing adequate airway and ventilation are basic, but fundamental parts of the management of all patients regardless of whether sedation, "light anaesthesia", or traditional day case general anaesthesia is provided.

The introduction of supra-glottic airways such as the laryngeal mask airway (LMA) has made a major contribution to expansion of day surgical anaesthesia.

7.1 **The laryngeal mask airway (LMA)**

The laryngeal mask airway was invented in 1983 by British anaesthetist, Dr Archie Brain. The LMA is a most useful alternative to achieve an adequate airway for most adult and paediatric patients during spontaneous breathing elective anaesthesia. The benefits of the LMA have become well established and much appreciated. The use of an LMA is associated with reduced need for opioid analgesics, e.g. decreased need for fentanyl/alfentanil, a less sore throat, and faster recovery compared with tracheal intubation. The end tidal gas concentration needed for accepting the LMA is lower than for the tracheal tub. The lower stress response for insertion and avoidance of muscle relaxation is also a well-acknowledged benefit of the use of an LMA. Most day case procedures do not require muscle relaxation, and avoidance of unnecessary use of relaxants is strongly recommended. Avoiding relaxation and promoting spontaneous breathing enables a better control of adequate depth of anaesthesia.

Neuromuscular blockade may of course be necessary to facilitate intubation or maintain muscle relaxation when needed for surgical reasons. Bad intubating conditions may cause pharyngo-laryngeal complications: the decision to avoid myorelaxants for tracheal intubation seems illogical when required. Today, however, there are a number of less invasive alternatives to intubation (e.g., supraglottic airways) that should first be considered.

The LMA is easy and atraumatic to insert, with minimal somatic and autonomic responses from the patient.

7.1.1 **LMA: a valid alternative to facemask and intubation**

The LMA is a suitable alternative to the facemask and to tracheal intubation in a wide variety of clinical situations.

As an alternative to the facemask, it provides hands-free anaesthesia and avoids potential episodes of impaired airway due to lack of attention from the attending anaesthetist.

As an alternative to intubation in elective anaesthesia, it provides patent airway without the stress of laryngoscopy or the need of muscle relaxation with associated risks.

A variety of re-usable LMAs is currently available and includes the following:

- LMA-Classic™
- LMA-Flexible™
- LMA-Unique™
- LMA-ProSeal™

Examples of an LMA–Supreme™ and an LMA–ProSeal™ are shown in Figure 7.1 a and b.

(a)

(b)

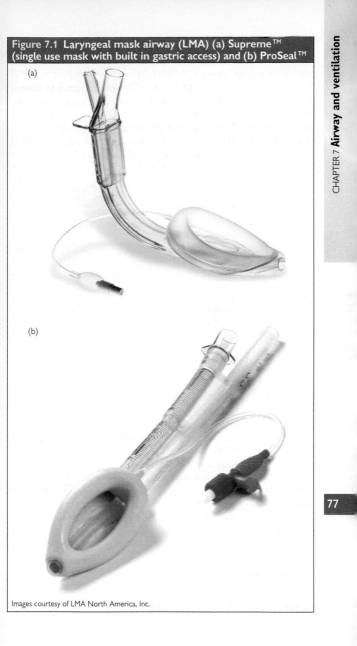

Images courtesy of LMA North America, Inc.

The LMA-ProSeal™ is a development of the LMA-classic intended to give better regurgitation protection and better seal during assisted/controlled ventilation. It has a bigger cuff and a canal for insertion of the gastric tube. It is therefore better suited for controlled ventilation.

7.1.2 LMA during laparoscopy

The use of the LMA during laparoscopic procedures has been debated for some time. There are still no prospective randomized and adequately powered studies that provide any clear answer. There is, however, increasing evidence of the use of LMA in laparoscopic surgery, lower as well as upper. These studies show that the LMA provides an acceptable airway and acceptable, and even good, operating conditions. Laparoscopic anaesthesia studies comparing a classic LMA to the ProSeal LMA have shown a favourable performance for the ProSeal. Both the classic LMA and ProSeal LMA have been shown to work efficaciously in suitable patients under laparoscopy receiving mechanical ventilation. Although there have been no cases of aspiration in these studies from its use during laparoscopy, the numbers are far too small to give a definitive answer as to its absolute safety.

7.1.3 LMA for open abdominal surgery

There is limited experience of the use of the LMA during open abdominal surgery. The experience is insufficient to make any firm comments.

7.1.4 LMA in special situations

The LMA has also been used successfully in the prone position in selected elective patients and has been shown to facilitate time to be ready for surgery. Changing position may, however, require control of the cuff pressure.

The LMA is a useful alternative during shoulder arthroscopy both when performed in the beach chair position or with the patient on his or her side.

Laryngeal mask airways have successfully been used in adenotonsillectomy. Surveys conducted in the UK and France have, however, shown that intubation is still most frequently used airway in tonsillectomy.

There is also recent positive experience from the use of the intubating LMA for microlaryngoscopy; a novel solution to a difficult procedure, which, with intubation, causes major haemodynamic challenges.

7.1.5 Summary

The LMA is today a widely accepted alternative airway during day case anaesthesia. It has become a most attractive alternative to an ordinary facemask as well as endotracheal intubation.

The advantages of the LMA are its ease of use, the fact that its use does not require laryngoscope or muscle relaxants, that it provides a safe airway for spontaneous or controlled ventilation, and that it is generally tolerated at lighter anaesthetic planes. The LMA does not, however, provide any guarantee for reflux/regurgitation and is therefore not recommended for non-fasted patients and/or for morbidly obese patients. There have been some case reports regarding aspiration during the use of an LMA in routine anaesthesia. The use of an LMA for laparoscopy should be made on an individual basis and any risk factor should be carefully sought and excluded (e.g., obesity) within adequate time without food and drink, or history of regurgitation. It should also be used with caution in patients with a history or signs of obstructive or abnormal lesions of the oropharynx.

7.2 Disposable LMAs

The single-use LMAs have been developed to a major extent in the light of the growing concern over reuse. Recent studies have indicated that despite stringent sterilization processes, the reusable silicone LMA has the potential for disease transmission through residual biological debris. The risks versus benefits should, however, always be put into perspective. The classical reusable LMA is a reliable airway with a low incidence of major complications and/or pharyngo-laryngeal morbidity. There have been an estimated 200 million patient uses of the LMA, over 2,500 academic papers related to its use and, some would argue, only one death directly attributable to its use. The LMA has been shown to be easy and simple to use and seemingly cost-effective as well as reassuringly safe in routine elective day case anaesthesia. There are today, however, a huge number of disposable LMAs available all with similar inflatable cuffs and shape. The disposable laryngeal mask is also to be placed blind, without the help of laryngoscope or other devices, in the hypo-pharynx.

7.2.1 Summary

Today a variety of single-use LMAs is available. There is no data showing major differences between the various disposable LMAs available.

7.3 Other alternative supra-glottic airways

A number of alternative supra-glottic airways have been introduced, as discussed below:

7.3.1 The cuffed oropharygeal airway (COPA)

The cuffed oropharyngeal airway (COPA) has been available for several years. There are several studies of its clinical use. It has been shown to be a acceptable alternative supporting free airway in elective anaesthesia.

7.3.2 **The Streamlined Liner of the Pharynx Airway (SLIPA)**

The Streamlined Liner of the Pharynx Airway (SLIPA) is another alternative supra-glottic airway with a reservoir. There are studies of its clinical use. It has been shown to be an acceptable alternative supporting a free airway.

7.3.3 **I-Gel airway**

The I-Gel airway (Intersurgical) is one of the latest in variety of alternative supra-glottic airways. It is a single-use supra-glottic airway without an inflatable cuff. The soft, elastomer-gel-made cuff mirrors the perilaryngeal anatomical structures. Theoretically, it is kept in place by adhesion forces as opposed to the conventional LMA, which seals by the pressure exerted to the perilaryngeal tissue. During the last few years several studies have been published of its clinical use. It has been shown to be an acceptable alternative airway.

7.3.4 **Summary**

Alternative supra-glottic airways are alternative disposables intended to provide a free airway. Much more evaluation from clinical practice and well-designed and powered studies is needed before their place in clinical practice can be fully evaluated. Most of the alternative supraglottic airways have been introduced with rather limited evidence of efficacy and safety. Some have been withdrawn and many have been modified. None have shown any clear and obvious advantage over the laryngeal mask airways.

7.4 **Intubation: tracheal tube**

The traditional oro-tracheal intubation is still the "gold standard" for securing the airway and to ascertain safe and effective ventilation in day case anaesthesia, and the recommended airway in emergent non-fasting patients. It should also be the technique of choice whenever there is risk of aspiration of gastric content or other fluids or material is at risk. The use of LMA during, e.g., tonsillectomy or adenectomy is still controversial.

Tracheal intubation is still generally seen as the technique for use in anaesthesia for laparoscopic surgery. There are a number of studies comparing the LMA to intubation. Most studies do not show any major adverse effect in either group of patients but in many studies one or a few patients require intubation due to inadequate airway control with the LMA. For laparoscopic anaesthesia, the ProSeal LMA seems to be a better option than the classic LMA and should be the supra-glottic airway of choice in cases where an LMA is assessed to be appropriate. Back-up intubation should, however, be readily available.

For day case anaesthesia, as for all anaesthetic service, a failed intubation/failed ventilation plan should be available.

7.4.1 **Summary**

- Securing airway and ventilation is of utmost importance in day case sedation/anaesthesia as elsewhere.
- Supra-glottic airways—the LMA—have made a major change in the practice of managing the airway in elective anaesthesia.
- The LMA has become the "gold standard" as a simple and safe alternative to both ordinary facemask and intubation in elective uncomplicated day case anaesthesia.
- The ProSeal LMA is used increasingly during anaesthesia for laparoscopy, but its use should be evaluated on an individual basis.
- There are a huge number of disposable LMAs available all with similar features to the classic LMA.
- There are also other supra-glottic airways available; their place in clinical anaesthesia needs further evaluation.

7.5 **Rescue plan for the management of the airway**

A rescue plan when the supra-glottic airway doesn't provide satisfactory airway and or secure ventilation should be in place. Intubation, although more invasive, should always be available as a back up in day case anaesthesia. There should also be a plan in place for failed intubation/management of free airway. Figure 7.2 shows a management plan for the "can't intubate ... can't ventilate" clinical scenario. Table 7.1 shows clinical features for different ways to secure the airway.

7.6 **Ventilation**

Minimizing the use of opioids and avoiding the use of muscle relaxants strongly promotes the possibility of spontaneous breathing. Spontaneous breathing should be the technique of choice in routine day case procedures. The LMA is also the most suitable for spontaneous breathing of prolonged duration. Assisted ventilation and occasional "alveolar recruitment manoeuvres" is recommended, especially in mildly obese patients, in order to counteract the formation of athelectasis.

Respiration should of course be monitored both with respect to SpO_2, and $EtCO_2$ and respiratory rate.

Spontaneous breathing on a LMA is also most feasible when having the patient on his or her side, in a "beach chair" during shoulder surgery, or when assessed to be acceptable in prone position.

Controlled ventilation may of course be an alternative when muscle relaxation has been deemed necessary. Assisted ventilation should always be instituted when inadequate ventilation becomes obvious, following induction and/or after opioid administration.

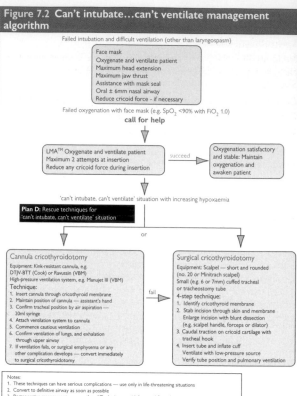

Figure 7.2 Can't intubate...can't ventilate management algorithm

Failed intubation and difficult ventilation (other than laryngospasm)

Face mask
Oxygenate and ventilate patient
Maximum head extension
Maximum jaw thrust
Assistance with mask seal
Oral ± 6mm nasal airway
Reduce cricoid force - if necessary

Failed oxygenation with face mask (e.g. SpO₂ <90% with FiO₂ 1.0)
call for help

LMA™ Oxygenate and ventilate patient
Maximum 2 attempts at insertion
Reduce any cricoid force during insertion

succeed →

Oxygenation satisfactory and stable: Maintain oxygenation and awaken patient

'can't intubate, can't ventilate' situation with increasing hypoxaemia

Plan D: Rescue techniques for 'can't intubate, can't ventilate' situation

or

Cannula cricothyroidotomy
Equipment: Kink-resistant cannula, e.g. DTJV-BTT (Cook) or Ravussin (VBM)
High-pressure ventilation system, e.g. Manujet III (VBM)
Technique:
1. Insert cannula through cricothyroid membrane
2. Maintain position of cannula — assistant's hand
3. Confirm tracheal position by air aspiration — 20ml syringe
4. Attach ventilation system to cannula
5. Commence cautious ventilation
6. Confirm ventilation of lungs, and exhalation through upper airway
7. If ventilation fails, or surgical emphysema or any other complication develops — convert immediately to surgical cricothyroidotomy

fail →

Surgical cricothyroidotomy
Equipment: Scalpel — short and rounded (no. 20 or Minitrach scalpel)
Small (e.g. 6 or 7mm) cuffed tracheal or tracheostomy tube
4-step technique:
1. Identify cricothyroid membrane
2. Stab incision through skin and membrane
   Enlarge incision with blunt dissection (e.g. scalpel handle, forceps or dilator)
3. Caudal traction on cricoid cartilage with tracheal hook
4. Insert tube and inflate cuff
   Ventilate with low-pressure source
   Verify tube position and pulmonary ventilation

Notes:
1. These techniques can have serious complications — use only in life-threatening situations
2. Convert to definitive airway as soon as possible
3. Postoperative management — see other difficult airway guidelines and flow-charts
4. 4mm cannula with low-pressure ventilation may be successful in patient breathing spontaneously

Figure 7.2 is reproduced with permission from the Difficult Airway Society.

Table 7.1 Clinical features for different ways to secure the airway

	Facemask	Laryngeal mask	ProSeal	Intubation
Easiness to use/insert	++	+++	++	++
Airway patency	+	++	++	+++
Airway protection	+	+	++	+++
Leak pressure	+	+(+)	++	+++

> **Box 7.1 Summary tips for setting up a day case anaesthesia service: the airway in day case anaesthesia**
>
> **Special demands**
> None, securing the patent and safe airway is one of most important parts in day case anaesthesia as well as elsewhere in anaesthetic practice.
>
> **Converting from an in-hospital to a day case program**
> Consider the use of a supra-glottic airway whenever feasible.
>
> **Setting up a hospital based freestanding day case service**
> Consider the use of a supra-glottic airway whenever feasible.
>
> **Think about**
> Is it possible to use a LMA? Promote Spontaneous breathing.

Further reading

Aziz L, Bashir K. Comparison of armoured laryngeal mask airway with endotracheal tube for adenotonsillectomy. *J Coll Physicians Surg Pak.* 2006; **16**: 685–8.

Blunt MC, Burchett KR. Variant Creutzfeldt–Jakob disease and disposable anaesthetic equipment-balancing the risks. *Br J Anaesth* 2003; **90**: 1–3.

Borkowski A, Perl T, Heuer J, Timmermann A, Braun U. The applicability of the ProSeal laryngeal mask airway for laparotomies. *Anasthesiol Intensivmed Notfallmed Schmerzther.* 2005; **40**: 477–86.

Brimacombe JR, Brain AIJ. *The Laryngeal mask Airway: A Review and Practical Guide.* WB Saunders, 1997.

Brimacombe JR, Wenzel V, Keller C. The proseal laryngeal mask airway in prone patients: a retrospective audit of 245 patients. *Anaesth Intensive Care.* 2007; **35**: 222–5.

Difficult Airway Management, edited by Dr Mansukh Popat., Oxford University Press, 2009.

Ecoffey C, Auroy Y, Pequignot F, Jougla E, Clergue F, Laxenaire MC, Lienhart A. A French survey of paediatric airway management use in tonsillectomy and appendicectomy. *Paediatr Anaesth* 2003; **13**: 584–8.

Gatward JJ, Cook TM, Seller C, Handel J, Simpson T, Vanek V, Kelly F. Evaluation of the size 4 i-gel airway in one hundred non-paralysed patients. *Anaesthesia.* 2008; **63**: 1124–30.

Gravningsbråten R, Nicklasson B, Raeder J. Safety of laryngeal mask airway and short-stay practice in office-based adenotonsillectomy. *Acta Anaesthesiol Scand.* 2008; Dec 6. [Epub ahead of print.]

Joshi GP, Inagaki Y, White PF, Taylor-Kennedy L, Wat LI, Gevirtz C, McCraney JM, McCulloch DA. Use of the laryngeal mask airway as an alternative to the tracheal tube during ambulatory anesthesia. *Anesth Analg.* 1997; **85**: 573–7.

CHAPTER 7 **Airway and ventilation**

Keller C, Brimacombe J, Bittersohl J, Lirk P, von Goedecke A. Aspiration and the laryngeal mask airway: three cases and a review of the literature. *Br J Anaesth.* 2004; **93**: 579–82.

Lange M, Smul T, Zimmermann P, Kohlenberger R, Roewer N, Kehl F. The effectiveness and patient comfort of the novel streamlined pharynx airway liner (SLIPA) compared with the conventional laryngeal mask airway in ophthalmic surgery. *Anesth Analg.* 2007; **104**: 431–4.

Lu PP, Brimacombe J, Yang C, Shyr M. ProSeal versus the Classic laryngeal mask airway for positive pressure ventilation during laparoscopic cholecystectomy. *Br J Anaesth.* 2002; **88**: 824-7.

Maltby JR, Beriault MT, Watson NC, Liepert D, Fick GH. The LMA-ProSeal is an effective alternative to tracheal intubation for laparoscopic cholecystectomy. *Can J Anaesth.* 2002; **49**: 857–62.

Natalini G, Lanza G, Rosano A, Dell'Agnolo P, Bernardini A. Standard Laryngeal Mask Airway and LMA-ProSeal during laparoscopic surgery. *J Clin Anesth.* 2003; **15**: 428–32..

Oczenski W, Krenn H, Dahaba AA, Binder M, El-Schahawi-Kienzl I, Jellinek H, Schwarz S, Fitzgerald RD. Hemodynamic and catecholamine stress responses to insertion of the Combitube, laryngeal mask airway or tracheal intubation. *Anesth Analg.* 1999; **88**: 1389–94.

Richez B, Saltel L, Banchereau F, Torrielli R, Cros AM. A new single use supraglottic airway device with a noninflatable cuff and an esophageal vent: an observational study of the i-gel. *Anesth Analg.* 2008; **106**: 1137–9.

Szmuk P, Ghelber O, Matuszczak M, Rabb MF, Ezri T, Sessler DI. A prospective, randomized comparison of cobra perilaryngeal airway and laryngeal mask airway unique in pediatric patients. *Anesth Analg.* 2008; **107**: 1523–30.

Thompson J, O'Neill S. Are supraglottic airways a safe alternative to tracheal intubation for laparoscopic surgery? *Br J Hosp Med (Lond).* 2008; **69**: 303.

van Zundert A, Al-Shaikh B, Brimacombe J, Koster J, Koning D, Mortier EP. Comparison of three disposable extraglottic airway devices in spontaneously breathing adults: the LMA-Unique, the Soft Seal laryngeal mask, and the Cobra perilaryngeal airway. *Anesthesiology.* 2006; **104**: 1165–9.

Vogelsang H, Uhlig T, Schmucker P. Severe multiorgan failure caused by aspiration with laryngeal mask airway *Anasthesiol Intensivmed Notfallmed Schmerzther.* 2001; **36**: 63–5.

Weksler N, Klein M, Rozentsveig V, Weksler D, Sidelnik C, Lottan M, Gurman GM. Laryngeal mask in prone position: pure exhibitionism or a valid technique. *Minerva Anestesiol.* 2007; **73**: 33–7.

Wilkins CJ, Cramp PG, Staples J, Stevens WC. Comparison of the anesthetic requirement for tolerance of laryngeal mask airway and endotracheal tube. *Anesth Analg.* 1992; **75**: 794–7.

Yano T, Imaizumi T, Uneda C, Nakayama R. Lower intracuff pressure of laryngeal mask airway in the lateral and prone positions compared with that in the supine position. *J Anesth.* 2008; **22**: 312–6.

Chapter 8

Postoperative nausea and vomiting (PONV): still "the little big problem"?

Key points

- Postoperative nausea and vomiting (PONV) is not only distressing but delays discharge; all efforts should be made to reduce its occurrence and to minimize the distress caused when it is experienced.

- PONV is a common problem after day case anaesthesia with a huge impact both on patient satisfaction and discharge/logistics.

- Risk-stratification and multi-modal prophylaxis should be administered accordingly.

- Triple prophylaxis has been shown to be effective although it does not entirely eliminate the risk in high-risk patients.

- All measures should be sought to provide adequate pain management with as little opioid administered as possible.

- Appropriate hydration, heart rate, and blood pressure should be secured.

- Even when all measures are taken there is still a risk in the high emetogenic group of patients.

- An adequately informed patient can without doubt be sent home while still experiencing PONV, as resting in the home environment is many times more satisfactory that in the day care facilities; Patients sent home with ongoing PONV should be informed how to act in case of prolonged symptoms beyond 48 hours.

The day case patient should be eligible for discharge within hours following the end of anaesthesia, and therefore postoperative nausea and vomiting (PONV) is not only a most distressing symptom, but a factor that delays discharge. Minimizing PONV is of outmost importance in day surgical anaesthesia and this can be done through the following:

- Risk stratification
- Basic prophylaxis
- Rescue therapy

Postoperative nausea and vomiting (PONV) continues to be the **"little big problem"** despite recent advances in anaesthesia. As the practice of surgery shifts toward short stay and outpatient treatment, the occurrence and management of PONV increases in importance due to its huge impact on delay of discharge. PONV also strongly contributes negatively to the patient's experience and thus to their level of satisfaction. There are several factors contributing to the occurrence of nausea and vomiting in the perioperative period. The most important factors should be evaluated in the preoperative assessment.

The simplified risk scores provide acceptable clinical discrimination and calibration properties compared with the more complex risk scores.

The simple PONV risk scoring should be done in advance and documented.

Female sex, non-smoking, history of motion sickness, and/or earlier experience of PONV and the need for postoperative opioids provide a basic list of major "risk factors"; risk factors for PONV are summarized in Figure 8.1.

There are, however, other factors with a major influence. Age (younger patients are far more susceptible to PONV than older patients), type of anaesthesia (general or other loco/regional), duration of anaesthesia (longer more than shorter), and type of surgery (breast surgery, gynaecological surgery, and ENT surgery far more than general orthopedic shoulder, or other) are also factors with independent influence on the risk of exhibiting PONV. A 10-year increase in age decreased the likelihood of PONV by 13%. A 30-minute increase in the duration of anaesthesia increased the likelihood of PONV by 59%. General anaesthesia increased the likelihood of PONV 11 times compared with other types of anaesthesia.

Sex, age, and sensitivity to motion and/or opioids cannot be changed. The impact of recent cessation of smoking is not well documented. It becomes obvious, however, that all measures necessary in order to eliminate and reduce the need for postoperative opioids should be sought. Pain management should as far as possible be based on non-opioid therapy. Duration of anaesthesia should cover the time needed associated with the procedure and prolongation due to any reason (e.g., unnecessary waiting times avoided). Avoiding general anaesthesia may be difficult but should be considered whenever possible. Loco-regional anaesthesia in combination with varying degrees of sedation should be considered. Pain may, for many procedures, be blocked by a regional or peripheral block, or just wound infiltration as for instance hernia repair. Loco-regional anaesthesia should be considered whenever feasible and if needed combined with light "conscious sedation", or when needed deeper sedation. Loco-regional anaesthesia in combination with adequate sedation is an alternative option to "full general anaesthesia". All means to reduce intraoperative opioids and unnecessary full general anaesthesia should be acknowledged. Loco-regional anaesthesia, in combination with any form of deeper sedation potentially having an effect on respiration, airway or protective reflexes, should be provided by anaesthesia personnel.

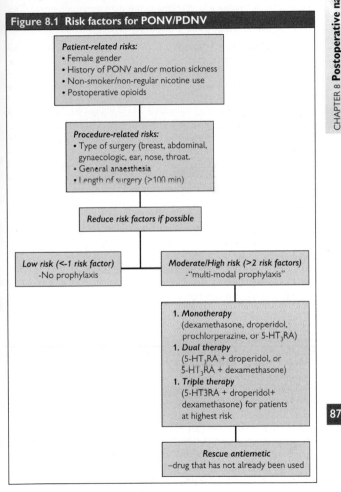

Figure 8.1 Risk factors for PONV/PDNV

Patient-related risks:
- Female gender
- History of PONV and/or motion sickness
- Non-smoker/non-regular nicotine use
- Postoperative opioids

Procedure-related risks:
- Type of surgery (breast, abdominal, gynaecologic, ear, nose, throat.
- General anaesthesia
- Length of surgery (>100 min)

Reduce risk factors if possible

Low risk (<-1 risk factor)
-No prophylaxis

Moderate/High risk (>2 risk factors)
-"multi-modal prophylaxis"

1. *Monotherapy*
   (dexamethasone, droperidol, prochlorperazine, or 5-HT$_3$RA)
1. *Dual therapy*
   (5-HT$_3$RA + droperidol, or 5-HT$_3$RA + dexamethasone)
1. *Triple therapy*
   (5-HT3RA + droperidol+ dexamethasone) for patients at highest risk

Rescue antiemetic
-drug that has not already been used

87

8.1 **Post-discharge nausea and vomiting (PDNV)**

Nausea and vomiting is not only experienced during the stay in hospital but also after discharge. Management of postoperative emesis includes both postoperative nausea and vomiting PONV while in the hospital environment, but also post-discharge nausea and vomiting (PDNV).

8.2 **Risk score gives advice about prophylaxis regimen**

A growing body of evidence suggests a multi-modal approach, a concept similar to that used for postoperative pain. Techniques for managing patients at high risk of developing PONV and PDNV are to administer a combination regimen that includes a 5-HT3-antagonist. No currently available regimen is entirely effective, however combining antiemetic agents from different drug classes is strongly recommended in order to minimize the risk, especially for high-risk patients. Because 5-HT3 receptor antagonists' dexamethasone and droperidol have different modes of action, their combination has been shown to reduce the risk of developing PONV or PDNV proportionally in the high-risk patient. Table 8.1 provides information regarding currently available antiemetic agents that are used in the treatment of PONV/PDNV.

The optimal doses are not known, dexamethasone or betamethasone 4–8 mg have been used in a many of studies documenting favourable effects. Low dose droperiodol, 0.5 to 1.25 mg has been studied extensively. Ondasetron in doses of 1 to 4 mg has been frequently used. Many studies suggest better effects from ondasentron when given at the end of surgery. Figure 8.2 shows the effects of dexamethasone, low dose droperidol, and ondasetron on PONV in high risk patients.

Table 8.1 Antiemetic agents		
Drug	**Adult Dosing**	**Adverse Effects**[a]
Phenothiazines		
prochlorperazine	5–10 mg iv at the end of surgery[b]	most common: sedation, lethargy, skin sensitization
	5–10 mg po before induction[b]	less common: cardiovascular effects, EPS, cholestatic jaundice, hyperprolactinemia
	25 mg rectally	rare: NMS, hematologic abnormalities
promethazine	12.5–25 mg iv at the end of surgery[b]	
	12.5–25 mg po before induction[b]	

Table 8.1 (Contd.)		
Drug	**Adult Dosing**	**Adverse Effects**[a]
Anticholinergics		
scopolamine	transdermal patch applied prior evening or 4 h before end of surgery[b]	most common: dry mouth, drowsiness, impaired eye accommodation rare: disorientation, memory disturbances, dizziness, hallucinations
Antihistamines		
dimenhydrinate	1–2 mg/kg iv	most common: sedation, dry mouth, constipation
hydroxyzine	25–100 mg im[b]	less common: confusion, blurred vision, urinary retention
Butyrophenones		
droperidol	0.625–1.25 mg iv at the end of surgery[b,c]	most common: sedation, hypotension, tachycardia
haloperidol	1–2 mg iv or im	less common: EPS, dizziness, increased blood pressure, chills hallucinations
Substituted benzamide		
metoclopramide	10 mg iv at the end of surgery[b]	most common: sedation, restlessness, diarrhoea, agitation, CNS depression less common: EPS (more frequent with higher doses), hypotension, NMS, supraventricular tachycardia (with iv administration)
Corticosteriods		
dexamethasone	4–10 mg iv before induction	most common: GI upset, anxiety, insomnia less common: hyperglycemia, facial flushing, euphoria, perineal itching or burning (probably secondary to vehicle and rate of injection)
Serotonin antagonists		
dolasetron	12.5 mg iv at the end of surgery[+] 12.5 mg iv rescue antiemetic[b]	most common: headache, asymptomatic prolongation of QT interval less common: constipation, asthenia, somnolence, diarrhoea, fever, tremor or twitching, ataxia, lightheadedness, dizziness, nervousness, thirst, muscle pain, warm or flushing sensation on iv administration
granisetron	0.35–1 mg iv at the end of surgery 0.1 mg iv rescue antiemetic[b,c]	

Table 8.1 (Contd.)		
Drug	**Adult Dosing**	**Adverse Effects**[a]
ondansetron	4–8 mg iv at the end of surgery[b,c] 1 mg iv rescue antiemetic	iv administration rare: transient elevations in hepatic enzymes
Neurokinin 1 antagonist		
aprepitant	40 mg po 1–3 h prior to induction of anaesthesia	most common: fatigue, hiccups less common: dizziness, headache, insomnia rare: transient elevations in hepatic enzymes

CNS = central nervous system; EPS = extrapyramidal symptoms; GI = gastrointestinal; NMS = neuroleptic malignant syndrome.

Data from Wilhelm S. Prevention of postoperative nausea and vomiting. *Ann Pharmacother* 2007; **41**: 68–78.

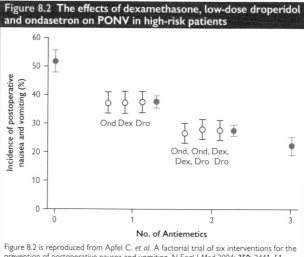

Figure 8.2 The effects of dexamethasone, low-dose droperidol and ondasetron on PONV in high-risk patients

Figure 8.2 is reproduced from Apfel C. *et al.* A factorial trial of six interventions for the prevention of postoperative nausea and vomiting. *N Engl J Med* 2004; **350**: 2441–51, © Massachusetts Medical Society. All rights reserved.

8.3 **Rescue therapy, when prophylaxis has failed**

Clinical data strongly suggest that rescue treatment is ineffective when the same drug used prophylactically is given. Therefore, rescue medications during the immediate postoperative period should be chosen from among drugs that have different mechanisms of action. For example, if ondansetron is administered for prophylaxis but PONV occurs, then promethazine or diphenhydramine could be given for rescue treatment rather than a repeat dose of ondansetron.

An algorithm for the management of PONV is provided in Figure 8.3.

8.4 **New options?**

The search for new agents is intense and the newest class of antiemetic agents is the NK-1 antagonists. Large studies with double-blind designs have been conducted to assess the effectiveness of the NK-1 antagonist aprepitant in the prevention of PONV.

Available data from these trials conducted to assess the effectiveness of the NK-1 antagonist aprepitant in the prevention of PONV as a single intervention have shown somewhat better effects than odansetron alone. Aprepitant was demonstrated to provide better nausea and emetic control than ondansetron 18–48 hours after surgery. The adverse effects of aprepitant treatment most commonly include pruritus, constipation, and nausea beyond 48 hours after surgery. Further studies are needed in order to better determine the place for aprepitant in clinical practice, as part of a multi-modal antiemetic strategy.

In patients at high risk of PONV, prophylaxis is strongly recommended. Also for PONV, a multi-modal approach has become the standard of care. Dexamethasone, low-dose droperidol, and one of 5-HT-3-antagonists have been shown to be more or less equally effective and additive when combined (see Apfel et al. [2004] and Figure 8.4). The effectiveness of metoclopramide is of a matter of dispute; however, low doses may exhibit minor added effect without any risk for major side effects.

Anaesthetic techniques have limited effects although propofol-based anaesthesia is generally recommended as the evidence for its superiority when looking at the entire postoperative course can be argued. Propofol-based anaesthesia is associated with a lower incidence of PONV in the early and intermediate postoperative period, but the effect is far less in the more protracted perspective.

Figure 8.3 An algorithm for the management of PONV

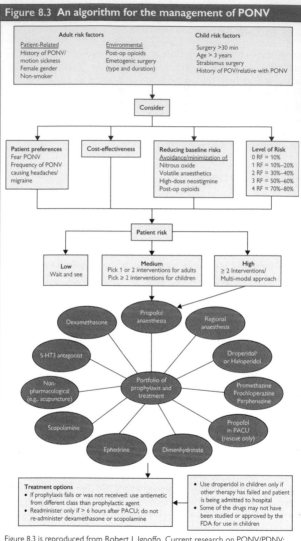

Figure 8.3 is reproduced from Robert J. Ignoffo, Current research on PONV/PDNV: Practical implications for today's pharmacist. *Am J Health-Syst Pharm.* 2009; **66**(Suppl 1): S19–24.

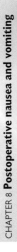

Figure 8.4 A factorial trial of six interventions for the prevention of postoperative nausea and vomiting

Figure 8.4 is reproduced with permission from Apfel C, et al. (2004) A factorial trial of six interventions for the prevention of postoperative nausea and vomiting. *The New England Journal Medicine*, **350**: 2441–51, © Massachusetts Medical Society. All rights reserved.

8.5 **Impact of high oxygen fraction**

The composition of fresh-gas has been discussed. Whether fresh gas flow consisting of high oxygen fraction could have an impact on the incidence of PONV has been a matter for discussion, but the evidence for any major effects is lacking. It has not been possible to support the significant effect of high FiO_2, (80% oxygen) in reducing PONV when analyzing the currently available documentation.

8.6 **Avoiding nitrous oxide**

Exchanging nitrous oxide with a high oxygen fraction may have a beneficial effect in anaesthesia for more extensive surgery. The independent effect of nitrous oxide during shorter day case anaesthesia seems more limited. When triple prophylaxis has been given, the independent effect of avoiding nitrous oxide seems very minor.

8.7 **Neostigmine: effect on PONV?**

The effects of neostigmine given for reversal of muscle relaxation have also been debated for some time. The clinical impact achieved from the use of clinical doses is, however, minimal. The benefit from adequate reversal of muscle relaxation (when needed) seems by far to outweigh the potential risk for PONV.

Administration of three or more prophylactic antiemetic agents has the most positive impact on emetic outcomes over 72 hours in patients at high risk of developing PONV. It is of importance to keep in mind that even with organizational PONV management guidelines, postoperative emetic symptoms and interference with patient functioning still occur in about 20% of high-risk patients.

8.8 **Rescue therapy**

In patients that have received PONV prophylaxis, it is advisable to rotate or select a drug from another class, for the treatment of PONV. It may therefore be an option not to use 5-HT-3 antagonists for prophylaxis, but to reserve these drugs for rescue therapy.

8.8.1 **Other supportive manuevers**

The emetic effects from vagal stimulation, low blood pressure should also be acknowledged. Adequate hydration and blood pressure control is of importance especially in susceptible patients.

Adequate hydration is also of importance. Intravenous administration of crystalloid 30 ml/kg to healthy women undergoing day-case gynaecological laparoscopy reduced the incidence of vomiting, nausea, and antiemetic use when compared with 10 ml/kg. Liberal use of intravenous fluids and prophylactic ephedrine in susceptible patients may help to reduce early postoperative fatigue and dizziness associated with the reduction in blood pressure during ambulation.

> **Box 8.1 Summary tips for setting up a day case anaesthesia service: postoperative nausea and vomiting (PONV)**
>
> **Special demands**
>
> PONV is a major concern in day case anaesthesia as elsewhere. Severe PONV is one reason for patients' dissatisfaction, delayed discharge and an increased risk for admittance to in-hospital care.
>
> **Converting**
>
> Every effort should be made to minimize the occurrence of PONV.
>
> **Setting up**
>
> All patients must be scored with regard to risk-factors for PONV and provided with prophylaxis accordingly.
>
> **Think about**
>
> Pain and PONV are the two of the most predominant factors influencing patients' satisfaction and patient turn around in day surgery.

Further reading

Ali SZ, Taguchi A, Holtmann B, Kurz A. Effect of supplemental pre-operative fluid on postoperative nausea and vomiting. *Anaesthesia* 2003 Aug; **58**(8): 780–4.

Apfel C. et al A factorial trial of six interventions for the prevention of postoperative nausea and vomiting *N Engl J Med* 2004; **350**: 2441–51.

Apfel CC, Kranke P, Eberhart I H, Roos A, Roewer N. Comparison of predictive models for postoperative nausea and vomiting. *Br J Anaesth.* 2002 Feb; **88**(2): 234–40.

Ignoffo RJ. Current research on PONV/PDNV: Practical implications for today's pharmacist. *Am J Health-Syst Pharm* 2009; **66**(Suppl 1): S19–24.

Magner JJ, McCaul C, Carton E, Gardiner J, Buggy D. Effect of intraoperative intravenous crystalloid infusion on postoperative nausea and vomiting after gynaecological laparoscopy: comparison of 30 and 10 ml kg(-1). *Br J Anaesth.* 2004 Sep; **93**(3): 381–5.

Orhan-Sungur M, Kranke P, Sessler D, Apfel CC. Does supplemental oxygen reduce postoperative nausea and vomiting? A meta-analysis of randomized controlled trials. *Anesth Analg.* 2008 Jun; **106**(6): 1733–8. Review.

Sinclair DR, Chung F, Mezei G. Can postoperative nausea and vomiting be predicted? *Anesthesiology.* 1999 Jul; **91**(1): 109–18.

Wilhelm S Prevention of Postoperative Nausea and Vomiting *Ann Pharmacother* 2007; **41**: 68–78.

Chapter 9

The recovery process and follow-up after day case anaesthesia

Key points

- Information and preparation of all aspects of the recovery process following discharge must be adequately secured in advance; anaesthesia and surgical stress as such cause profound inabilities in retrieving information after completion of the procedure.

- The goal is not only to ascertain adequate intraoperative quality, patient- and surgeon-wise, but also to have a rapid and safe recovery. The use of a multi-modal analgesic and anaesthetic technique aims to facilitate the recovery process, enabling patients to become eligible for discharge within hours after the end of surgery.

- Pain management and avoidance of postoperative nausea and vomiting (PONV) and general fatigue is of utmost importance; it is of huge importance that all personnel have the mindset to facilitate the recovery and coach the early mobilization process.

- Patient information, written and oral, covering all aspects of the postoperative course should be provided.

- Postoperative medications should be prescribed preoperatively and available at home.

- Transport and escort for the journey home should be planed. Generally, patients should not be discharged without an escort after general anaesthesia, regional anaesthesia, monitored anaesthesia or sedation; caregivers need to verify a safe ride home.

- Driving after ambulatory surgery in general anaesthesia cannot be considered safe until the next day, 24 hr postoperatively.

- Information about what to do in the case of complications or questions should be provided.

- Some form of quality assurance programme and follow-up should be present; evaluation of major morbidity, return to hospital visits, and patients' satisfaction with the programme are all quality measures that should be evaluated on a regular basis.

Recovery after day case anaesthesia follows the same pattern as for anaesthesia in general. The patient scheduled for day case surgery is, however, to be discharged within hours after end of anaesthesia/surgery. **Proper information and preparation for all aspects of the recovery process following discharge must be adequately secured in advance.** Not only all anaesthetics, but also the surgical stress involved cause profound disabilities in retrieving information following surgery/anaesthesia.

The postoperative information should cover all aspects of the recovery and rehabilitation process; pain medication, wound care, rehabilitation programme, and any special information (e.g. need for antibiotics, additional wound dressing changes, etc.)

It is strongly recommended that prescriptions for medications are all provided in advance in order to make it possible to have medication available on the patient's return home. Alternatively, patients should be provided with take-home medication in order to manage for at least 24 hours.

All pain medications including rescue analgesics should be available when the patients come home. In high risk patients antiemetics should also be provided to take at home. The surgeon should have determined the need for antibiotic and or thromboprophylaxis before surgery in accordance with accepted routines and made these available at before discharge.

9.1 **The recovery process**

The recovery process can be separated into several different stages, including:

- emergence;
- discharge eligible;
- street fit.

9.1.1 **Emergence**

The early recovery of consciousness and vital functions, the "emergence", is traditionally evaluated by the Aldrete score (see Table 9.1). Day case anaesthesia patients often regain an adequate Aldrete score within minutes following cessation of anaesthesia administration. Patients commonly regain vital signs and consciousness in the operating theatre `and can safely by-pass stage I recovery. Fast tracking, bypassing the traditional recovery room going to stage II recovery, has become increasingly popular after short day case anaesthesia.

Table 9.1 Post-anaesthesia discharge scoring system (PADSS)	
1	**Vital signs** 2 = Within 20% of preoperative value 1 = 20–40% of preoperative value 0 = 40% of preoperative value
2	**Ambulation and mental status** 2 = Oriented × 3 and has a steady gait 1 = Oriented × 3 or has a steady gait 0 = Neither
3	**Pain, or nausea/vomiting** 2 = Minimal 1 = Moderate 0 = Severe
4	**Surgical bleeding** 2 = Minimal 1 = Moderate 0 = Severe
5	**Intake and output** 2 = Has had PO fluids and voided 1 = Has had PO fluids or voided 0 = Neither

The total score is 10. With patients scoring ≥ 9 considered fit for discharge home.

9.1.2 Discharge eligible

Discharge eligible is the second stage frequently evaluated by discharge scores (e.g., Chung modified discharge score; see Table 9.2).

Simple stand, walk, drink and void tests are far more pragmatic and easy to use. Secure adequate pain in accordance with set limits (generally < 4 out 10 on the visual analogue scale (VAS) and no or mild nausea is also of importance to achieve before leaving the hospital.

Discharge from the day surgical unit is, however, not being street-fit, but merely able to continue the more protracted recovery phase in the home environment. It is strongly advised that patients at discharge should have an escort during transfer to home and also at home during the initial postoperative phase. Patients should be strictly informed not to drive or use complex machinery or perform other tasks that demand full cognitive skill within 24 hours after day case anaesthesia. After minor procedures in local anaesthesia and sedation more rapid regain of cognitive function has been shown. Still it seems advisable from a medico-legal perspective to recommend avoidance of driving until the next day.

Table 9.2 A modified postanaesthesia discharge scoring system (MPADSS)	
1	**Vital signs** 2 = Within 20% of preoperative value 1 = 20–40% of preoperative value 0 = 40% of preoperative value
2	**Ambulation** 2 = Steady gait/no dizzness 1 = With assistance 0 = None/dizziness
3	**Nausea/vomiting** 2 = Minimal 1 = Moderate 0 = Severe
4	**Pain** 2 = Minimal 1 = Moderate 0 = Severe
5	**Surgical bleeding** 2 = Minimal 1 = Moderate 0 = Severe
The total score is 10. With patients scoring ≥ 9 considered fit for discharge home.	

9.1.3 **Both anaesthetic and surgical considerations**

Many decisions include both anaesthetic and surgical considerations. The unit must develop clear routines that are structured and transparent for the decision processes associated with the care of the day surgical patient. Discharge/eligible for discharge status should be decided not only based on anaesthetic considerations, but should also take surgical aspects into account. In order to maintain safety and to avoid jeopardizing the surgical intervention discharge, information about rehabilitation and sick leave are aspects that need to be addressed by the responsible surgeon.

9.1.4 **Street fit**

"Street fit" or back to basic activities of daily living is the third and most important stage of recovery, when the patient can resume normal activity; go back to full time work without interference from residual effects of the anaesthesia, analgesics, and surgery; and without procedural-related interference. Residual effects from anaesthesia are in most cases minimal after 24 hours. Potential effects of pain medication on cognitive function and general well being must, however, be taken into account.

Return to work and duration of sick leave is in most institutions the general responsibility of the surgeon. Length of hospital stay should not per se influence the duration of sick leave.

It is important to provide patients with oral and written information about what to do in case of "emergencies". Both patient and escort should be provided with a phone number and information on how to act if re-admission is required for some reason.

9.1.5 Follow-up, evaluate, update the programme and then once again...

Some institutions make pro-active follow-up phone calls to patients 1–2 days after surgery not only in order to provide support and guidance, but also in order to gain feedback. Many surgeons see the patient on an outpatient visit. However, structured follow-up and registration of minor and/or major complaints and complications are uncommon.

Morbidity and mortality in ambulatory surgery is rare, and thus the patient's quality of life (i.e., the ability to resume normal activities after discharge home) should be considered to be one of the principal end-points after ambulatory surgery and anaesthesia. There is, however, no standard developed measure used to evaluate patient satisfaction with anaesthesia care. Further study should be conducted to develop standardized instruments to measure this outcome.

In recent years, a shift has occurred toward patient-centred study outcomes such as quality-of-life questionnaires. There is, however, no fully validated technique currently available for this outcome.

These end-points, outcome of anaesthesia and surgery, are most certainly interrelated but not identical. As an example, although there are data suggesting that improved postoperative analgesia leads to better patient outcomes, there is insufficient evidence to support subsequent improvements in patient-centred outcomes such as quality of life and quality of recovery.

Keeping track of complications related to surgery as well as anaesthesia should be done on a regular base. Follow-up of quality of care and patients' satisfaction should be done at least intermittently in order to gain insight into the performance of the programme. Increase of complications and/or complaints about the quality of care should prompt analysis of the programme and bring changes accordingly. Figure 9.1 outlines a process of continuous improvement which can be applied to the day case anaesthesia unit.

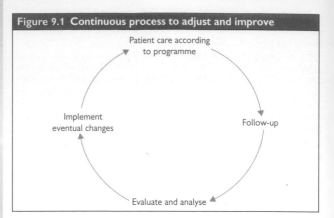

Figure 9.1 Continuous process to adjust and improve

Patient care according to programme

Follow-up

Evaluate and analyse

Implement eventual changes

Box 9.1 Summary tips for setting up a day case anaesthesia service: the recovery process and follow-up after day case surgery

Special demands

The day case patient is to leave the hospital within hours after the end of anaesthesia.

Converting

Emphasize the mindset of providing adequate intraoperative anaesthesia; but team efforts to gain rapid mobilization and ambulation.

Setting up

Mindset, all personnel should be aware of and work for good and adequate quality of care but with the goal of rapid mobilization and ambulation.

Think about

Pain, nausea and vomiting and fatigue are common factors delaying discharge. Actions should be taken to avoid or minimize the occurrence of these symptoms.

9.2 Looking to the future

Standardization, production and the maintenance of quality of care

Day case surgery is becoming increasingly popular and more and more procedures are done on a short-stay basis. However, shortening a hospital stay must not jeopardize safety or quality of care.

Planning, structuring and logistics are fundamental parts of day case surgery. Much of the pioneering work in day case surgery has now become well-established and a gold standard not only in day case practice but also increasingly in hospital care.

Day case surgery should continue to develop safe and effective medical care. It has become increasingly popular to implement standardized process/management systems. Many day case centres have implemented ISO standards in order to fully subscribe to 'Industrial process oriented logistics and quality systems'. Similarly, many centres have also adopted 'lean production' thinking in order to facilitate the entire process. Day case anaesthesia should be a natural part of this process and an effective oriented environment, but should nevertheless maintain **safety and quality of care** as its first priority.

Finally, the bases for day case anaesthesia practice remain: adequate preoperative assessment and information, professional and evidence-based anaesthesia, multi-modal pain and PONV management, and clear and structured discharge criteria and rescue/feedback planning.

Further reading

Awad IT, Chung F. Factors affecting recovery and discharge following ambulatory surgery. Can J Anaesth. 2006 Sep; **53**(9): 858–72. Review.

Chanthong P, Abrishami A, Wong J, Chung F. 471577—patient satisfaction in ambulatory anesthesia: a systematic review. Can J Anaesth. 2008 Jun; **55** Suppl 1: 471577.

Chung F. Discharge criteria—a new trend. Canadian journal of anesthesia [0832-610X] 1995 **42**(11): 1056.

Chung F, Assmann N. Car accidents after ambulatory surgery in patients without an escort. Anesth Analg. 2008 Mar; **106**(3): 817–20.

Herrera FJ, Wong J, Chung F. A systematic review of postoperative recovery measurements after ambulatory surgery. Anesth Analg. 2007 Jul; **105**(1): 63–9.

Kluivers KB, Riphagen I, Vierhout ME, Brölmann HA, de Vet HC. Systematic review on recovery specific quality-of-life instruments. Surgery. 2008 Feb; **143**(2): 206–15. Epub 2007 Dec 21. Review.

Liu SS, Wu CL. The effect of analgesic technique on postoperative patient-reported outcomes including analgesia: a systematic review. Anesth Analg. 2007 Sep; **105**(3): 789–808. Review.

Index

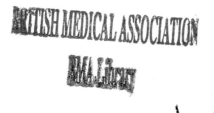